MEDICINAL PLANTS
AND
GLOSSARY OF SELECTED TERMS

MEDICINAL PLANTS AND GLOSSARY OF SELECTED TERMS

B. S. DESAI
F.M. PARABIA
Y.T. JASRAI
M.H. PARABIA

BHARATIYA KALA PRAKASHAN
DELHI (INDIA)

First Published : 2007

***Published by* C.P. Gautam**
BHARATIYA KALA PRAKASHAN
3421-A, IInd Floor, Narang Colony, Tri Nagar,
Delhi-110035. Phone : 27393083,32967505 (O)
E-Mail : bkp3421@yahoo.co.in

ISBN : 978-81-8090-145-4

Laser Type Setting by
A-ONE GRAPHICS
Pitampura, Delhi-110088

Printed By :
BDH Printer at Salasar Imaging Systems
Delhi.

Dedicated

To

Late Acharya Shri Bapalal G. Vaidya.

FOREWORD

The word Ayurved is derived from the Sanskrit root **Ayu** (life) and **Veda** (knowledge), in essence, **the Science of Life.** It is most ancient indigenous system of medicine, dating back to the vedic ages (1500-800 BC).

In India ever since Aryan civilization sprang into prominence, people started worshipping natural elements. Yajurveda deals extensively with rituals and various plants used in rituals. Atharvana veda exclusively deals with medicinal uses of plants, diseases and their treatments. Ayurveda, a branch of Atharvana veda is regarded as an Upa-veda, which is the most ancient and scientific treatise on medicine and disease.

Medicinal plants constitute one of the worthiest gifts of nature to the mankind India has a rich heritage of medicinal plants diversity as well as the knowledge system based on medicinal plants. Though Ayurveda depends upon plants to a large extent, almost all other systems of medicine also use plants as their basic resource.

The quality of a drug depends on the quality of the raw material and the genuineness of the material. Besides, the plant resources also face problems of over-exploitation, extinction adulteration, unhealthy processing, storage and identification etc.

The compilation on **Medicinal Plants and Glossary of Selected Terms** including related information is of great importance in present scenario. I must compliment the authors for such a painstaking task for the benefit of students, researchers and all those interested in the field of medicinal plants and their management.

—Dr. Parimal H. Trivedi
Vice-Chancellor
Gujarat University,
Ahmedabad-380009

LIST OF ILLUSTRATIONS

CONTENTS

PROLOGUE

"Trees are imperfect men." – Emerson.

Vedas have worshipped forests and trees." 'Aryas' used medicinal plants (Rigveda). The word "Medi-herbs" leads to the thought of miraculous and super natural cures.

The ancient "Aryan sanskrity" is based on harmony with 'aranya' (Forests). Our poets too have highly held 'Forest and Trees'. This is evident from the classics like 'SHAKUNTAL', 'KUMARSHAMBHAVAM', 'RAGHUVANSHAM'. Inspite of rich flora and ancient literatures we remained complacent and gradually ignored Ayurveda. Allopathic Drugs dominated.

During last few decades; since researches have taken momentum, ethnomedicinal claims are tested, reported world over. People are now keen to know about plants and their medicinal uses. Bioproducts and biodiversity's importance is well recognized and also accepted as science. Worldwide forest products turnover was almost 3000 million dollars in year 2000. India's contribution was merely 2 %. Informations on electronic medias, books, new reports are not within the reach of common man. Besides lot of controversies exist so as to correct identification, classification and vernacular (local) names. Keeping this in mind this book is written with utmost care to make people informative with facts.

Prof. Govindachari has rightly stated:

"To be willing to learn from living traditions of any great culture, one has to drop, one's prejudices, modify one's world views and attitudes and assume a discriminate receptiveness".

Therapeutic wisdom of a culture is a dynamic experience base that demands a close participation for understanding and learning. One most important approach can be the pragmatic utilization of demonstrated therapautic wisdom to relieve human sufferings, not withstanding the scientific understanding of the underlying mechanisms.

In this book widely used drugs and those, which are approved, generally are included.

Book is a compilation of Latin names, Sanskrit names, Gujarati, Marathi and Hindi names of medicinally important plants. Their properties and uses are given alongwith information on safety aspects and Bio-activities wherever available. This book is mainly for those who wish to begin the study of Medicinal- plants. Some interesting informations on ayruvedic weights & measures, various ayurvedic formulations terminology and reference books, are compiled and presented.

B. S. Desai.
F. M. Parabia
Y. T. Jasrai.
M. H. Parabia.

INTRODUCTION

In the history of evolution plants and other animals preceded man. However, since the advent of man all the species started evolving together. Man being the superior species, affected the environment, many a times influenced evolutionary, processes of many species (e.g. cultivated plants), helped conserving species long destined to be extincted (e.g. *Ginkgo biloba*) or caused extinction of many species (Dodo, Passenger Pigeon) etc. Man out of his 'sapiens' employed quite a few of the plant species as food and medicine.

Hindu culture – the ancient Aryans – appear to be quick in recognizing the medicinal value of local plants, animals and mineral resources. The treatment to their ills were offered through panchkarma, diet control and modification, medicines and surgical corrections too. The knowledge system of Ayurveda – the science of life had flourished well. But as it has happened with many ancient systems, the Ayurveda also suffered through some inherent social and political customs and interventions.

The first blow to surgical science was affected by the advocates of "non-violent - Ahinsa". As this belief in Ahinsa received political asylum (rajyashrya), the surgical teachings and the dissections of corps were banned. Of course, this led to the development of alchemy (rasa sashtra) during the jain regimes in India.

The social custom affected the further development of Ayurveda. This effect began somewhere in seventh century with muslim invasion and lasted through 20th century. One could surmise two factors, 1. Operation of Intellectual Property Right (IPR) and 2. The suppression of local intellects by the foreign rulers. It will not be utterly out of place to elaborate on these two factors.

1. Operation of IPR

The Arabic and European travellers were greeted well by the Indian natives. This also facilitated the free exchange of knowledge between the native scholars and the versatile travellers. But when they came to India first as conquerer and then as rulers, the Indian scholars withdrew themselves into a protective shell. They grew extremely reticent. The flow and the continuity of knowledge from generation to generation dried up. The sagas mostly withheld their knowledge in absence of "proper pupil" (supatra). In one way or other the practice was to safe guard the IPR, by limiting the spread of information and knowledge.

2. Suppression of Local Intellects by The Foreign Rulers

Indian system suffered the most under the 200 years of British rule. This is the period when all branches of science witnessed exponential pace of development. The Indian science was ruthlessly subjected to humiliation and rejection. Ayurveda was no exception. We lost the touch with the classical Sanskrit, the language in which our knowledge was preserved.

The educational system created novel philosophers. The knowledge system was so designed, that it conditioned the minds of our scholars against indigenous knowledge. The renovations, refreshments and progress are the crux of any science. Ayurveda suffered and stagnated.

Independent India is once again witnessing the revival of age-old practice of herbology. The people at large wish to know more about the cultural heritage. Many of them seek refuge in ayurvedic system of treatment for their dreaded diseases. Herbalists were all botanists once upon a time. The era of specialization separated them as two distinct schools of experts. The present day botanists hardly know about the medicinal properties of the plants and the herbal medicinal practitioner can hardly identify plants correctly!

Nonetheless, authors feel that the current time is once again showing signs of integration. Present book is an initial step to provide an interface so as new researcher can develop enough preliminary insight to carryout research in medicinal plants. The information contained in this book is a kind of compilation gathered from the scattered literature on Ayurveda and medicinal plants in the regional languages of the country.

It is hoped that, it can serve as a handbook to the workers and students of medicinal plants, botany, pharmacy and other applied aspects.

ABBREVIATIONS

1.	IPR	:	Intellectual property Right
2.	B and H's	:	Bentham and Hooker's System of Classification
3.	R and D	:	Research and Development
4.	BARC	:	Bhobha Atomic Research Centre, Mumbai
5.	BSI	:	Botanical Survey of India, Kolkatta
6.	CAZRI	:	Central Arid Zone Research Institute, Jodhpur
7.	CCRAS	:	Central Council for Research in Ayujrveda and Siddha, New Delhi
8.	CCRH	:	Central Council for Research in Homeopathy, New Delhi
9.	CCRUM	:	Central Council for Research in Unani Medicine, New Delhi
10.	CDRI	:	Central Drug Research Institute, Lucknow
11.	CIMAP	:	Central Institute of Medicinal and Atomatic Plants, Lucknow
12.	CPCRI	:	Central Plantation Crops Research Institute
13.	CSIR	:	Council for Scientific and Industrial AResearch
14.	DCOMPWB	:	Directorate of Cinchona and other Medicinal Plants, Govt. of West Bengal
15.	FRI	:	Forest Research Institute
16.	FRLHT	:	Foundation for Revitalization of Local Health Traditions
17.	ICAR	:	Indian Council of Agriculture Research
18.	ICMR	:	Indian Council of Medical Research
19.	IICB	:	Indian Institute of Chemical Biology
20.	IIHR	:	Indian Institute of Horizontal Research
21.	IIT	:	Indian Institute of Technology
22.	MOEF	:	Ministry of Environment and Forests

23. MOHFW : Ministry of Health and Family Welfare
24. DBT : Department of Biotenchnology
25. DST : Department of Science and Technology
26. NBRI : National Botanical Research Institute
27. NBPGR : National Bureau of Plant Genetic Resources
28. NCL : National Chemical Laboratory
29. NII : National Institute of Immunology
30. RRL : Regional Research Laboratory
31. TBGRI : Tropical Botanic Garden and Research Institute
32. TFRI : Tropical Forest Research Institute
33. UNESCO : United Nations Educational Scientific and Cultural Organization
34. WHO : World Health Organizaton
35. GAP : Good Agricultural Practice
36. GMP : Good Manufacturing Practices.
37. GC : Gas Chromatography
38. GLC : Gas Liquid Chromatography
39. GSC : Gas Solid Chromatography
40. HPLC : High Perfoemance/Pressure Liquid Chromatography
41. HPTLC : High Performance Thin Layer Chromatography
42. UV : Ultraviolet
43. IR : Infrared
44. AAS : Atomic Absorption Spectrophotometer
45. DNA : Deoxyribosa Nucleic Acid
46. PCR : Polymerase Chain Reaction

Chapter–1

WEIGHTS AND MEASURES IN AYURVEDA

Weights and Measure: Conversion Tables

In ancient books old measurements are mentioned as 'Rati', 'Masa', Tola etc. Now, we should be aware of their conversion in metric system as given below:

One Rati			=	121.5 mg
Two Rati			=	243.0 mg
Six Rati	= one 'anabhar'		=	729 mg
Eight Rati	= one 'masabhar'		=	972 mg (could be rounded upto 1000mg =1g)
Twenty four Rati	= three 'masabhar'	=four anabhar	=	2.920 g =3g
Ninety six Rati	= twelve 'masabhar'	= one tolas	=	11.66 g =12g
Four tolas			=	46.66 g
10 tolas			=	116.64 g

Measurement for Liquids

One taral gram	=	1 ml water
Half ounce	=	14 ml
Eight ounce	=	227 ml
Twenty ounce	=	570 ml
Twenty four ounce	=	682 ml

Weights And Measures Conversion Factors

1 Grain	=	0.06489 g
1 g	=	24 wheat grains
2 Anna	=	1.5 g

4 Prastha	= 256 tolas
4 Prastha	= 3072 g
8 Rati =1 Masha	= 1000 mg
1 Rati	= 121 mg
96 Rati =12 Masha	= 12 g
1 Pavli	= 3 g
1 Rupee	= 12 g
1 Rupee	= 32 Val
4 Val =2 Annas	= 1.5 g
2 Jav	= 1 Habba
3 Habba	= 1 Kirat
2 Wheat	= 1 Chanothi
	= 1 Rati
	= 121 mg
3 Chanothi	= 1 Val
20 Wheat	= 1 Kherooti
3 Kherooti	= 1 Drachm.
1 Drachm	= 1 (3/7) Dirram.
	= 4 g
	= 1 dang.
	= 7/40 Miskal.
1 Miskal	= 4111 Masa.
3 Drachm	= 1 Tola.
	= 12 g.
1 Tola	= 12 Masa.
2.5 Rupees =7.5 Miskal	= 30 g.
4 Annas	= 1 Pavli.
2 Pavli =1 Ardho	= 1 Gadianu.
2 Gadianu =1 Tola	= 12 g.

1 Gadianu	=	6 g.
18 Rai (mustard) =3 Jav	=	2 Wheat.
6 Chanothi	=	1 Anna.
12 Chanothi =1 Masa =24 wheat	=	1 g.
1 Masa	=	1 g.
1 Ounce =2.5 Tola	=	30 g.
8 Tola	=	1 Pal.
40 Tola	=	1 Sheer.
2 Sheer	=	1 Prastha.
32 Sheer	=	1 Dron.
5 Tola	=	1 Navtank.
2 Navtank	=	1 Pasheer.
2 Pasheer	=	1 Ardhosheer.
40 Sheer	=	1 Mann.
32 Val =1 Tola	=	12 g.
1 grain	=	0.0648g.
1 Dirram	=	4 g.
1 g.	=	24 Wheat grains.
1 Wheat grain	=	40 mg.
1 Masa =1 g.	=	12 Chanothi.
1 Val	=	3 Chanothi.
4 Val	=	12 Chanothi.
1 g.	=	4 Val.
1 Val.	=	250 mg.
1 Rupee	=	32 Val.
1 Rupee	=	8 g.
½ Rupee	=	4 g.
¼ Rupee	=	2 g.

2 Aani =1 g.	= 4 Val.
8 Paise	=1000 mg.
1 Paise	=125 mg.

Antidotes

Drugs	**Antidotes**
Afin (Opium)	Sakar
Tobacco	Milk
Chanothi	Dhana and Milk
Jher Kachola	Ghee and to induce vomiting
Hirakasi ($FeSO_4$)	Butter milk
Shilajil	Ghee
Raskapoor	Cow milk
Bhilamo	Badam, Til (Tal)
Kapoor	Kesar

Chapter–2

PLANT GROUPS AND INGREDIENTS

Some Important Drug Groups

Astavarga	=	Meda, Mahameda, Jivak, Rushbhak, Kakoli, Kshirkakoli, Ruddhi and Vruddhi.
Panchamrut	=	Galo, Musli, Sunth, Gokhru, Shatavari.
Eklavan	=	Shindhav.
Panchvalka	=	Vad, Piplo, Pipli, Umardo and Paras piplo.
Kshirvruksh	=	Umbaro, Vad, Pipal, Paras piplo, Galo.
Chaturbeej	=	Methi, Asaliyo, Kali jiri, Ajmod.
Dashmool	=	5 Laghu panch mool +5 Guru panch mool.
Triphala	=	Harde, Baheda, Amla.
Trikatu	=	Sunth, Mari and Lindi peepar.
Trimad	=	Vavding, Nagarmoth, Chitrakmool.
Trisam	=	Harde, Sunth and Galo.
Triloh	=	Sonu (gold), Rupu and Copper.
Panchosan A	=	Lindipeepar, Peeprimool, Chavak, Chitrak and Sunth.
B	=	Harde, Ajmo, Sanchal, Hing, Sunth.
Bala Chatushtaya	=	Bala, Mahabala, Atibala and Nagbala.
Panchmool.		
(i) Laghu Panchmool	=	Salvan, Pithvan, Ringani, Ubhi ringani and Gokhru.
(ii) Guru Panchmool	=	Bili, Shivan, Tentu, Patala and Arni.
(iii) Baladimool	=	Baldana, Satodi, Mrudagparni, Masparni and Arand.
(iv) Gokshuradi	=	Gokhru, Bordi, Indravarni, Kasundri and Sirish.

(v) Shatavaryadi = Shatavari, Vidari, Jivanti, Medhasinghi, Jivak.

Dasmool- made up of ten roots are as follows:

1. Aegle marmelos. = Bili.
2. Gmelina arborea. = Shivan.
3. Desmodium gangeticum. = Salvan, Shaliparni.
4. Oroxylum indicum. = Tentu, Shyonak.
5. Premna serretifolia/Clerodendrum multiflorum. = Agnimanth, Arni.
6. Pseudarthria viscida/Uraria picta. = Pithvan.
7. Solanum xanthocarpum. = Bhoyringni.
8. Solanum indicum. = Brihati, Ubhiringni.
9. Strereospermum suaveolens. = Patala.
10. Tribulus terrestris. = Gokshur, Gokhru.

Guggal- Guggal or Guggul is a resinous gum exudating from Commiphora Wightii (Arnott.) Bhandari. – Shrub belonging to family Burseraceae. The Plant dies after the gum is extracted. Raw guggal is used only as incense. For the preparation of oral medicines Guggal needs to be purified. Guggul is never used alone. It is considered as Yogvahi (a catalyst, may be).

The basic guggul, therefore is Triphala-Guggul. Raw Guggul is boiled with Triphala-Quath. On softening, the Guggul is beaten hard with pestle or a hammer and immersed again in Triphala Quath. The process is extremely cumbersome. It is repeated till the guggul dissolves in quath. Quath is then filtered through cloth to remove debris. Quanth is boiled again till a thick consistency is achieved. The final lump is rolled into pills or pressed into the tablets. The basic purified guggul,thus obtained is used in the preparation of about 40 different medicines. A few of them are listed below.

(A) Amrita guggal : Galo, Guggal, Triphala, Trikuta, Vidang, Dalchini, Nashotar. Used in Gout and rheumatism.

(B) Dashang guggal : Sunth, Pippali, Chitrak, Triphala, Nagar moth, Vidang, Guggal. Effective in obesity.

(C) Kishor guggal : Triphala, Guggal, Galo, Trikatu, Vidang, Nashotar, Ghee. Specifically used in Gout.

(D) Kanchnar guggal : Kanchnar bark, Triphala, Trikatu, Elaichi, Dalchini, Guggal. Used in Scrofula and enlargement of lymph glands, tumours and thyroid disfunctioning.

(E) Mahayogaraj guggal : Panchkol, Hing, Ajmod, Sarsav, Jeera, Indrajav, Patha, Vidang, Kutaki, Ativish, Bharangi, Vacha, Triphala, Guggal, Abhrak, Ras-sindur. Used in neuromuscular diseases, rheumatism, fibrositis and gout with Rasnadiquath.

(F) Punarnava guggal : Satodimool, Arand-mool, Sunth, Guggal, Arand oil, Nashotar, Danti-mool, Galo, Triphala, Chitrak, Sindhav, Vidang, Swarna-makshik bhasma, Punarnava churna. Used in Gout, rheumatism and sciatica.

(G) Shiva guggal : Triphala, Arand mool/oil, Guggal, Gandhak, Vidang, Pippali, Dantimool, Sunth. Useful in rheumatism, sciatica, constipation and amoebic dysentery.

(H) Swayambhu guggal : Bavchi, Shilajeet, Guggal, Swarna makshik-bhasma, Loha-bhasma, Gorakh mundi choorna, Triphala, Karanj leaves, Khadir-sar, Galo, Vacha, Nashotar, Danti-mool, Jaiphal, Haldar, Parad (Hg).

(I) Trayodashang guggal : Keekar fruit, Ashwagandha, Galo, Hafushu, Shatavari, Gokhru, Rasana, Valiyari, Ajmod, Sunth, Guggal, Ghrit (ghee). Used in sacral pain, sciatica and nervous system related diseases.

(J) Vatari guggal : Erand taila, Gandhak, Guggal, Harde, Baheda, Amla, Ajmod, Jeeru, Vidang, Devdaru Useful in rheumatism.

(K) Yograj guggal : Guggal, Chitrak, Pippali mool, Ajmod, Jiru, Vidang, Devdaru, Elaichi, Sindhav, Rasna, Gokhru, Dhana, Triphala, Moth, Sunth, Pippali, Dalchini, Khus, Yavakshar, Talis-patra, Taj. Useful in rheumatism and Menorrhagia.

Important Tips

(A) Fresh plants are advisable, but vavding, lindi peepar, gol (Jaggery), dhana, honey and ghee better be one year old.

(B) Galo, kadoo bark, vasa, shatavari, aswagandha and valiyari should be fresh while utilizing.

(C) Normal dose for Kastha aushadha (Churna) is 5 g, unless otherwise mentioned.

(D) Herbal medicines can also have poisonous effects. Therefore, dose alteration and self medication should be avoided.

(E) Asav, gold, bhasmas and ras-sindur etc., are rasayanas and useful even if older.

(F)

Patients	**Contra indicated formulations**
Anaemic	Mercury
Pregnant lady	Asalio, Cinchona, Arecanut and Aghedo.
TB	Somal containing drugs
Hyper Acidity	Bhallatak

Ayurvedic Medicines- Are of three types.

Animal Origin : Honey, milk, ghee (also works as mediators) bones, horns.

Plant Origin : Medicinal Plants.

Mineral Origin : Gold, Arsenic, gems, etc.

Rushies

They were having awareness of potency and storage of plants. For this let us look at the instructions given in Charaka Kalpasasthan I and II, "Herbs should be stored in houses with doors opening to the east or to the north and storage room should be windless, fire-resistant, moisture-free and dust proofed."

Properties, uses and applied researches in medico botany are based on health and ayurveda so let us examine briefly definations.

Ayurveda- Ideal defination would be a science that is with "the science times of life" and about life. As a science it would be open to change and growth (B.G. Vaidya).

Health- Results from worldview of a harmonious working of body, mind and soul. According to Sushruta "one, whose three doshas, digestion, seven tissue functions, metabolism, excretion are balanced and that whose senses, mind and spirits are cheerful that one is called healthy". Charak also has a similar defination of health and diseases as- "The abnormal state of body tissues and functional system is called disorder and their harmony is natural health". In Ayurveda, happiness (sukha) is Health and misery (Dukhah) is disease/disorder. From above now let us have look at technical defination of Ayurveda, which states that, "Where in beneficial and adverse influence leading to health and disease are described and quantified". In short "The state of physical, mental and spiritual well being is health".

Important Aspects of Ayurveda

Nidan : Diagnosis based on tridoshas i.e. Vata, Pitta and Kapha.

Poorvaroopa : Pre-clinical form of functional biochemical disorders.

Roopa : Clinical symptoms.

Upashaya : Diverse therapeutic modalities of diet, remedies etc.

Samprapti : Disease taxonomy and detailed information, understanding of doshas is most vital for diagnosis as well as for uses of medicinal plants (their effect on doshas).

Qualities of drugs viz rasa (taste), guna (physical/chemical properties), veerya (metabolic property), vipaka (metabolite taste), and prabhava (potency) are basis of management of disease in Ayurveda. RASA plays important role as follows:

Vata Dosh is relieved by sweet, sour and salty rasa but is aggravated by bitter, spicy and astringent rasa.

Pitta Dosh is relieved by sweet, bitter and astringent rasa but is aggravated by sour, salty and spicy rasa.

Kapha Dosh is relieved by bitter, spicy and astringent but is aggravated by sweet, sour and salty rasa.

Vipaka of sweet, sour and spicy retain same taste whereas vipaka of salty is sweet and that of bitter is spicy.

Gunas of medical drugs are related to density, viscosity and dispersibility – very important in relation to bioavailability.

Rasa, guna, veerya, vipaka and prabhav: any material used as medicine is described for its five properties expressed after administration to the patient.

Prabhav is the unique pharmacodynamic property of a material used as medicines.

Chapter–3

HERBAL DRUG PREPARATIONS

According to charaka drug differs with respect to land, season, source, flavour, taste etc and also sufferers (who differs with respect to weight, age, vitality and state of disease).

Mehods of Herbal Drug Preparation

In ayurveda, drug administration is known as "Bhaishajya Kalpana". Following are the methods of herbal drug preparation and raw material processing.

1. **Quath (Decoction):**
   - ❑ This is the most basic method in Ayurveda. Drug is soaked in water at proportion of 1: 16, 1: 8 or at 1: 4 and boiled till ¼ remains. For boiling earthen vessel is recommended.
2. **Anupam and Yogvahi (Adjuvants):**
   - ❑ Anupam is the way of drug administration, which increases the effect of the drug: e.g; water, milk and honey.
   - ❑ Yogvahi is an adjuvant taken with the medicine for better effect.
   - ❑ E.g. Sugar, honey, black pepper, salts like Table salt, Rock salt (Sindhav), Black salt (Sanchal), Guggal (gum), Trikatu (Ginger +Pepper + Long Pepper), Jeeru, milk, ghee, jaggery, oil, cow's urine (Gawmutra), Vinegar, alcohol etc are used as Yogvahi.
   - ❑ Jeeru is used in cough, acidity and as pitta shamak medicine.
   - ❑ Trikatu is given in indigestion.
3. **Sheet Kashaya (Cold infusion):**
   - ❑ Mix-drug +Hot water at 1: 2 ratio and keep for over night. Next morning filter and consume the liquid.
4. **Fant (Infusion):**
   - ❑ Pour hot boiling water on a fine powder of drug at 1: 2 ratio. Keep for 2 minutes. Allow to cool and consume the mixture.
   - ❑ E.g. Sudarshan Churna is a compounded drug of 38 plants, all contain bitter principles recommended for fever, is best if administered as fant.

5. Swaras (Self Extract):

- ❑ Reduce the fresh drug into paste and then express the juice while pressing in the cloth.

6. Kalk:

- ❑ Fine paste of fresh plant or a plant part.

7. Paniya:

- ❑ Watery extract of drug in water at ratio of 1: 64. Boiled till half remains. Filter, cool and consume.
- ❑ E.g. Chukuvallum, best for cold and cough, is the form of drinking- water-decoction, traditionally used in Kerala.

8. Kshir Pak (Milk decoction):

- ❑ Drug 1 part: milk 2 parts: water 2 parts, boil till 2 parts of water is totally evapourated and only drug +milk remains.
- ❑ Principle is that, the drug is cooked with the milk; water is added because on boiling milk becomes thicker and heavy to digest, and many drugs do not cook well, if boiled only in milk.
- ❑ E.g. Arjun Churna is given as heart tonic after making its Kshirpak.

9. Bhavana:

- ❑ It is for increasing the concentration of soluble parts to increase the potency of the drug.
- ❑ Add juice of the same fresh material while properly levigating.
- ❑ When liquid dries add again fresh juice, repeat the same procedure, to eliminate fibers and water, only soluble contents are increased.
- ❑ Amalaki Rasayana has 21 bhavanas of Amala swarasa.
- ❑ Arogya Vardhini has bhavana of Neem bark decoction.
- ❑ Aloe vera juice is frequently used to treat the Bhasmas (Metal oxides). This detoxifies metal.

10. Putpak:

- ❑ Fresh material is wrapped in Ficus benghalensis leaves; this in turn is wrapped in fine cloth smeared in fine clay.
- ❑ First dry in sun and put in fire.
- ❑ Fire by dung cake or agro waste is called 'put'. Cool it, then remove dried mud and cloth.
- ❑ Take out the cooked drug with leaves, crush with leaves. Extract the juice and use the juice.

11. Kanji (Fermented Starch):

- ❑ This is one of the Anupan.

- ❑ Flour of grain (Barley, Jawar, Bajara), take 1: 24 with water.
- ❑ Store it in bottle or in earthen vesicle. Tie with cloth so insect does not enter.
- ❑ Put in dark for 4-6 days till sourness is developed.
- ❑ Filter and throw away the residue.
- ❑ Liquid is Kanji used as anuupan, recommended in women's problems.

12. Arnal (Fermented Rice):

- ❑ Rice 1: 48 water.
- ❑ Cooked, after cooking stir it vigorously.
- ❑ Store in airtight glass vessel for about 7 days. This arnal is given as anupan.

13. Tushamb/Tushnodak:

- ❑ Roast whole grains of barley with husk and powder. Mix at 1: 24 with water.
- ❑ Leave for 6-7 days for fermentation.
- ❑ Filter, the liquid is Tushamb.

14. Sauvir:

- ❑ Whole barley grains are cooked and mixed with 24 parts of water and stored in glass bottle till gets sour.

15. Asava and Arishtha:

- ❑ Ferment of fresh juice of uncooked drug is asava. E.g. Drakshasav, Arjunasav.
- ❑ Ferment of decoction of the same is arishtha, prepared in off season, when dried material is used, so first cooked and then used. E.g. Arjunarishtha.
- ❑ 1 litre of extract (juice or decoction)
- ❑ 250 g sugar
- ❑ 10 g whole wheat
- ❑ Activated yeast.
- ❑ In earlier days when yeast was not available, natural cultures were provided by the flower of "Dhatki" (Woodfordia Ifalies). Finally whole vessel is covered with cloth and allowed to stand for 4 weeks.
- ❑ Stir the solution once a day to mix sugar and yeast.
- ❑ May add Citric acid, which prevents bacterial contamination, yeast uses Citric acid also as food.
- ❑ After 4 weeks, decant.
- ❑ Add preservatives like, sodium benzoate and bottle.

Drugs are considered to be of two kinds

- Promotive of vigour
  - Virilitic (helps for positive health, immunity and to restrict ageing for health).
  - Rasayan (Vitalizer) (helps to replenish vital tissue constituents
- Curative of disease

For good formulations, standardization and accuracy both are equally important. Correct dosage is vital to avoid harmful effects.

Chapter–4

CONSTITUTION OF SELECTED AYURVEDIC MEDICINES

Arishtas and Asavas

Fermented product of decoctions is called "ARISTHA".

When an aqueous extract is fermented, it is called "ASAVA".

(A) Abhyarishta : Harde, Draksha, Vidang, Mahuda, Gokhru, Nashotar, Dhana, Dhataki-flowers, Indruvarni, Soya, Sunth, Dantimool, Moch rasa (simlo) (uses – cholagogue, constipation, dyspepsia, piles).

(B) Amritarishta : Galo, Dashmoola, Jeera, Pitpapdo, Saptaparni bark, Trikatu, Nagarmotha, Nag-kesar, Katuki, Ativish, Kadoo, Ativish, Indravarni (useful periodic fever).

(C) Ashokarishta : Ashok bark, Dhatki-flowers, Jeeru, Nagarmoth, Sunth, Daru haldi, Ambahaldar, Rose, Triphala, Vasa, Chandan, (uses- leucorrhoea, menorrhagia, uterine trouble).

(D) Dashamularishta : Dashmula, Chitrak, Pushkar-mool, Lodhra, Galo, Amli, Vijayasar, Manjistha, Devdaru, Vidang, Bharangi, Behda, Satodi, Jatamanshi, Sariva, Kali-jiri, Rasna, Nisoth, Pippali, Haldi, Nagkesar, Nagarmoth, Indrajav, Dalchini, Elaichi, Kasturi.

(E) Khadirarishta : Khadir, Triphala, Daruhaldar, Bavchi, Dhatakiful, Kankol, Lavang, Jaiphal, Dalchini, Kesar, Mari, (uses- Leprosy, skin diseases, cardiac problems).

(F) Kutjarishta : Kutaj, Draksha, Dhataki-phool (dysenteries).

(G) Arvindasava : Kamal, Khas, Manjishtha, Elaichi, Bala, Jatamansi, Nagarmoth, Sariva, Harde, Baheda, Vacha, Amla, Nisot, Patol, Pit-papdo, Arjun bark, Madudo, Jethimadh, Draksha, Dhataki-flowers (Used as tonic for children).

(H) Lodhrasava : Lodhra, Pushkarmool, Elaichi, Vidang, Triphala, Ajmod, Indrajav, Kariatu, Kutki, Bharangi, Tagar, Chitrak, Pippali-mool, Patha, Indrajav, Nagkesar, Kutaj, Moth, Honey (useful in urethritis, cystitis leucorrhoea, dysmenorrhoea, endo-metritis, anaemia, piles, sprue).

(I) Kumariasava : Dashmool, Pushkar-mul, Chitrak, Galo, Harde, Lodhra, Amla, Tandaljo, Manjistha, Behda, Pipar (Chava), Kushta, Mulethi, Kothi, Devdaru, Vidanga, Pippali, Bharangi, Ashtavarg, Jeera, Supari, Rasna, Nagod, Shringi, Haldar, Jatamansi, Nagarmoth, Sariva, Vasaka, Shatavari, Indravarni, Nagkesar, Satodi, Kumarpathu, Lavang, Kankol,

Safed-chandan, Mari, Javantri, Tamalpatra, Akal-karo, Jaiphal, Kavach, Ajmod, Ghodavaj, Bala, Sunth, Dhana (Cures hepatitis, Infantile Liver Cirrhosis).

(J) Lohasav : Loha-bhasma, Mari, Sunth, Pipali, Triphala, Ajmod, Vidanga, Moth, Chitrak, Honey (Digestive tonic, Anaemia, Dropsy, Piles, Chronic fevers).

Choorna

Is to be taken with honey or water best when used. Fresh upto six months after collection. Dose: about 5g two to three times a day.

(A) Ajmodadi : Ajmo, Mochrasa, Sunth, Dhatki-ful (diarrhoea).

(B) Ashwagandhadi : Ashwagandha, Galo, Satavari, Dashmoola, Bala, Ati-bala, Pushkarmool (tonic).

(C) Avipattikar : Trikatu, Triphala, Nagarmoth, Tamal-patra, Sindhav, Lavang, Vidang, Elaichi, Nasotar, (Acidity, Heart burn, hypochlorhydra).

(D) Gangadhar : Bilapulp, Moch-rasa, Patha, Dhatki-ful, Dhana, Manjishtha, Sunth, Motha, Ativish, Afin, Lodhra, Dadam, Kutaj bark, Gandhak, Paro (Amoebic dysentery).

(E) Gokshuradi : Gokhru, Talimkhana, Shatavari, Kavanch, Nagbala, Ati-bala (Aphrodisiac, diuretic, nervine tonic).

(F) Narayana Churna : Harde, Ajmod, Dhana, Triphala, Kali-jiri, Pippali, Jira, Trikatu, Vidang, Danti-mool, Nasotar, Indravarni, Ghodavaj, Sapta-parni. (Gastric troubles).

(G) Saraswat : Kustha, Ashwagandha, Sindhav, Ajmod, Jira, Kali-jiri, Sunth, Mari, Pippali, Patha, Shankh-pushpi, Vacha, Brahmi-rasa.

(H) Shringyadi : Katori (dabhi), Shringi, Sunth, Mari, Harde, Baheda, Amla, Bharangi, Pushkarmool, Panchlavan (Hic-cough, asthma, cough) with warm H_20.

(I) Sudarshan : Triphala, Bhoy-ringni, Haldar, Trikatu, Pippali-mul, Galo, Morvel, Dhamaso, Kutaki, Pit-papdo, Motha, Bala, Limbdo, Pushkar-mul, Jethimadh, Kutaj, Ajmod, Indravarni, Bharangi, Dalchini, Gulab, Khas, Chandan, Ativish, Shalparni, Vidanga, Tagar, Chitrak, Devdaru, Mari, Patol, Jeevak, Karmal, Kakoli, Talis-patra, Kariyatu (All types of fever).

(J) Swadishta Virechan Churna : Jethimadh, Shat-puspi, Gandhak, Sounf , Sugar (purgative, in piles, for fissure) with hot water.

(K) Vaishwanar : Sindhav, Ajmo, Sunth, Harde. (Rheumatism and rheumatic heart, carminative).

(L) Navayasa Loha : Trikatu, Triphala, Moth, Vidang, Chitrak, Lohabhasma (jaundice, anaemia).

(M) Vadwanal : Shindhav, Pippali, Pippli mool, Long peeper, Chitrak, Sunth, Harde (Appetizer, Digestive).

Avelha Orleha

is a marmalade in all its essentials, fortified with different herbs.

(A) Chavayan Prash : Bilva, Agnimantha, Kambari bark, Bala, Shalparni, Mashparni, Pippali, Gokhru, Kakdasinghi, Bhoi-amla,

Draksha, Jeevanti, Pushkar-mool, Agar, Haldar, Galo riddhi, Jeevanti rishbhak, Kachur, Motha, Ativish, Punarnava, Meda, Elaichi, Chandan, Kamal- pushpa, Vidari, Kakoli, Kaknasika, Amla, Pippali, Dalchini, Taj, Nagkesar (Alterative tonic).

Quath

Means decoction prepared by boiling drugs in water (should be used within twelve hours of preparation).

(A) Abhayadi : Harde, Nagarmoth, Dhana, Rakta-chandan, Kamal, Vasa, Indravaruni, Galo, Patha, Sunth, Kutki, (fevers, delirium and complications).

(B) Amritadi : Galo, Vasa, Patol, Nagarmoth, Sapta-parni, Khadir, Neem leaves, Harde (Fever, urticaria, skin diseases).

(C) Bharangyadi : Galo, Nagarmoth, Devdaru, Sunth, Pippali, Bharangi, Pushkar mool (Cough and fever).

(D) Brihat manjishtadi : Manjishtha, Kutaj-bark, Galo, Motha, Kateri, Sunth, Harde, Neem, Patola, Kutaki, Bharangi, Vidang, Devdaru, Indravarni, Bhangro, Pipali, Patha, Shatavari, Khadir, Triphala, Kariyatu, Ashwagandha, Vasa, Pit-papdo, Anantmul, Ativish (blood purifier, skin diseases).

(E) Patoladi : Patol-mool, Mulethi, Kutki, Harde, Devdaru, Mamiro, Haldar, Chandan, Dantimool, Indrajav, Pippali (Fever, antacid, indigestion).

(F) Rasnadi Panchak : Rasna, Erand mool, Shatavari, Sanchar, Vasa, Galo, Devdaru, Ativish, Harde, Patha, Sunth, (Rheumatism).

(G) Arakadi quath : Ankdo, Pipali-mool, Daru-haldi, Mari, Nagod, Pippali, Rasna, Bhangro, Satodi, Chitrak, Vacha, Kariyatu, Sunth (Pneumonia, malarial fever).

Herbo-Mineral As pills (Tablets)

(A) Chadraprabha Vati : Vidanga, Chitrak, Trikatu, Triphala, Long-peeper, Devdaru, Kariyatu, Pippali-mool, Moth, Vacha, Swarna makshik-bhasma, Harde, Shindhav, Yavakshur, Rasna, Ativish, Shilajeet, Guggal, Loha bhasma, Sugar, Nasotar, Jaiphal (Piles, fistula, gonorrhoea and urinary trouble).

(B) Agnitundi Vati : Parad, Gandhak, Ajmod, Vidang, Vishtinduk, Palashbeej. Administered with Moth quath. (Flatulence, Indigestion, bed wetting).

(C) Arogya Vardhini : Parad, Gandhak, Loh-bhasma, Abhrak-bhasma, Tamra (copper) bhasma, Triphala, Shilajeet, Guggal, Chitrak, Kutaki (Aperient, dropsy, anorexia, jaundice, liver cirrhosis).

(D) Chintamani : Parad, Gandhak, Abharak bhasma, Loha bhasma, Shilajeet, Chandi bhasma, (Rajat) swarna bhasma, Bhringraj swarasa, Chitrak quath, Arjun quath (pulmonary cardiac tonic, with wheat quath).

(E) Kumar kalyan : (with swarna muktha), Rasa sindur, Swarna bhasma, Abharak bhasma, Mukta bhasma, Loha bhasma, Swarna makshik bhasma (tonic for children).

(F) Makardhwaj : Gold leaf, Parad, Gandhak, Kumari-rasa, Kapur, Lavang, Jaiphal, Kasturi (Alterative and general tonic).

(G) Sarvatobhadra : Swarna bhasma, Rajat bhasma, Loha bhasma, Abharak bhasma, Shilajeet, Gandhak, Swarna makshik bhasma, Varun quath (chronic renal pains and renal T(B)

(H) Soota shekhar rasa : Parad, Swarna bhasma, Trikatu, Dhantura seed, Gandhak, Tamra bhasma, Shankh bhasma, Bilva pulp, Bhringrasrasa (Acidity, vomiting, indigestion, colic, heart burn).

(I) Vasant Kusumakar : Swarna bhasma, Rajat bhasma, Vang bhasma, Seesa bhasma, Kant loha bhasma, Abhrak bhasma, Praval bhasma, Mukta bhasma, Cow milk, Vasa, Kamal rasa, Kasturi, (Diabetes) with ghee and honey.

(J) Swarna vasant malti : Swarna bhasma, Mukta bhasma, Hing, Kalimirch, Kapur bhasma, Butter, Nimbu rasa, (chronic debiliting fever, cough, rehabilitation of T. B. patient) with Pippali churna and honey.

(K) Vatvi dhwansa : Parad, Gandhak, Nag bhasma, bang bhasma, Loha bhasma, Tamra bhasma, Abhrak bhasma, Pippali, Sunth, Trikatu quath, Triphala quath, Chitrak rasa, Akalkar rasa, Nagod rasa, Dhatri rasa, Abhrak rasa, Nimbu rasa (neuralgia, colic, joint pains and nervous disease).

(L) Yogendra : Rasa sindoor, Swarna bhasma, Kanta loha bhasma, Abhrak bhasma, Mukta bhasma, Kumari rasa (General and nervine tonic).

(M) Shilajitwadi : Shilajeet, Abhrak bhasma, Swarna bhasma, Loha bhasma, Guggal, Bhringraj rasa, (spermortorrhoea).

(N) Trayoshnadi Mandur : Trikuta, Triphala, Moth, Vidanga, Chavya, Chitrak, Daru haldi, Swarna makshik bhasma, Pippali mul, Devdaru-churna, Mandoor-churna (Anaemia, jaundice, dropsy).

Taila (Oil)

medicated oil prepared in sesamum (Tal) oil, used externaly and/or for massage.

(A) Mahavishgarbha tail : Til oil, Dhantura root, Nagod, Satodi, Erandmool, Ashwagandha, Chitrak, Bhangro, Neem bark, Ishwari, Dashmul, Shatavari, Anantmul, Gorakhmundi, Vidari, Apamarga, Bala, Nagbala, Mahabala, Vasa, Galo, Kustha, Moth, Devdaru, Panchlavan, Jiru, Indrajav root (Sciatica, tinnitus, nervous diseases).

(B) Narayan : Shatavari, Shalparni, Vacha, Errand, Kateli, Karanj root, Atibala, Milk, Satodi, Devdaru, Soya, Chandan, Tagar, Elaichi, Jatamansi, Ashwagandha, Sindhav, Rasna (anginal, pleuritic and rheumatic pain).

Lavan

is prepared by packing herbs with salt in an earthen pot in airtight condition and burnt with dung cake.

(A) Bhaskar : Pippali, Pippali mool, Dhana, Kali-jiri, Sindhav, Talispatra, Nagkesar, Sanchal, Mari, Sunth, Dalchini, Elaichi, Dadam bij (Indigestion, flatulence and loss of appetite).

(B) Mandoor : Mandoor, Baheda, Cow's urine, Shindhav (Anaemia) with honey.

Rasavaidak

drugs of mineral origin frequently treated with herbs.

(A) Abhrak : Mica.

(B) Ambar : Sham digested visceral content of whales. (Debility).

(C) Kadikhar : Silver nitrate ($AgNO_3$).

(D) Kant loha : Iron.

(E) Kapariyu (S.karpur) : Calamine, zinc carbonate (S-kharpur) by-products of mines.

(F) Gandhak : Sulphur (purified only) (Appetiser, digestive, anthelmintic, useful in skin diseases).

(G) Chhipla : Oyster shell made up of $CaCO_3$ (Osteroporosis).

(H) Jasat : Zn (zinc).

(I) Navsar : Ammonium chloride (NH_4Cl) (Pain hysteria).

(J) Parad (Hg) : Mercury.

(K) Alum (Fatakadi) : Potassium or ammonium aluminium sulphate (Vomit and fever).

(L) Manahshila : Mansi (Reatgar), Red Arsenic Sulfide. If unpurified leads to debility (constipating, urinary diseases and diabetes).

(M) Shilajeet : Shilajeet (Asphalt) (Renal diseases, diabetes, leucorrhoea). Jew's pitch, (silaras). It is a mass or substance ejected from rock crevices in the lower Himalayas during hot weather, composed of gummy matrix (dark red) and of bitter taste having four types as follows- 1.Gold (red colour); 2. Silver (white); 3. Copper (blue colour); 4.Iron. (blackish brown). Last one is widely used in medicines.

Property : Antiseptic, antiphlogistic, alterative, laxative, tonic, expectorant, diuretic and lithotriptic.

Uses : Jaundice, enlarged-spleen, diabetes, dyspepsia, piles, indigestion, renal calculli, epilepsy, insanity, gynec problems, tuberculosis, R.T.I., aneamia and neurasthenia.

(N) Shankh : Ocean product (Splenomegaly, diarrhoea).

(O) Shankh Jiru : One kind of stone (Silicate of magnesia) (Menorrhagia, wounds).

(P) Swarna Makshik : Sonamukhi (Iron pirites) (Anaemia, jaundice, slow fever).

(Q) Swarna : Gold.

(R) Somal (S-pasan) : Oxide of arsenic (Ringworm, black spot on skin).

(S) Sindur (Red lead) : By-metal of lead.

(T) Kasim : Hirakasi : $FeSO_4$ (Anemia, TB, spleen enlargement, pain).

Astavarga : Eight tubers known as astavarga used in chyavanprash.

Uses : As revitaliser

Following are the tentative representative suggested as Astavarga.

1. Jivak : *Malaxis wallichii* (Orchidaceae)
2. Rishbhvak : *Malaxis muscifera* (Orchidaceae)
3. Kakoli : *Fritillaria roylei* (Liliaceae)
4. Kshir kakoli : *Lilium polyphyllum* (Liliaceae)
5. Mahameda : *Polygonatum verticillatum* (Liliaceae)
6. Meda : *Polygonatum cirrhifolium* (Liliaceae)
7. Ridhhi : *Habenaria edgeworthii* (Orchidaceae)
8. Vriddhi : *Habenaria latilabris* (Orchidaceae)

Chapter–5

MATERIAL PREPARATION

Material and the Preparation where it is used

Material		Preparation
Adu (Sunth)	:	Rasnadi kwath, Chandra prabhavati, Soubhagya sunthi, Goksuradi guggal, Parpatyadi kwath
Afin	:	Afinasav, Dugdhavati, Arkadi choorna, Mahavatari-ras.
Agnimantha	:	Dashmoolarist.
Ajmod	:	Ajmodadi choorna, Agnitundivati.
Amla	:	Chavyanprasa, Brahma-rasayan, Dhatriloha,Triphala, Agnitundivati, Sanjivanivati, Amritask kwath, Hingastak churna, Amritaskarista, Lavan bhaskar churna, Agani tundi vati,
Anantmool	:	Sarivadi kwath, Sarivadyasav.
Ankdo	:	Arkadi qwath, Arkadi taila.
Ardusi (Vasa)	:	Vasaka churna, Vasakarist, Vasaka kwath.
Arjun	:	Arjunaristha, Arjuntwak-choorna.
Asok	:	Asokarista.
Asthavarga	:	Chavyanprasa.
Asthishrinkala	:	Ashthi-sanghar taila. (Hadsankal)
Aswagandha	:	Ashwagandhadi choorna, Ashwagandharista, Ashwagandha Rasayan.
Ativish	:	Ativisadi choorna, Balchatur bhadraras, Amritrista, Vatsayadi quath.
Baheda	:	Triphala, Talisadi-churna, Lanvangadivati, Sudarsan churna, Agnitundivati, Punarnavamandur,
Bala	:	Baladi kwath, Baladyaristh, Chandanbala-lakshadi taila, Sudarshan churna.
Bans (Bamboo)	:	Sitopaladi churna, Chandraprabhavati, Talisyadi churna, Sudarsan churna.
Baval (babul)	:	Lavangadi vati.
Bavchi	:	Vidanga lepa.

Bharangi : Bharangyadi kwath, Sudarsan-churna, Shringyadi-churna, Yograj guggal.
Bhilamo : Sanjivani vati, Amritabhallatok.
Bhoy Ringani : Kantkarighrita, Kantkari-avleha, Chavyanprash Dasmoolaristh, Sudarsan churna, Shringyadi churna.
Bhoy Amli : Sudarshan churna, Dashmularista, Brihatyadi kwath.
Bhringraj : Bhringraj taila, Bhringraj spirit.
Bijoru : Rasonavati, Agnitundivati.
Bili : Bilva-panchakqwath, Bilwadi-churna, Dashmularista, Gangadhar churna.
Brahmi : Brahmi grhita.
Chameli : Jatiyaditaila, Jatiyadivati, Jatiputradi kwath.
Chandan : Chandanadi vati, Chandanadi choorna, Sudarshan Churna, Pipplyasav.
Chitrak : Chitrakadi churna, Amalayasdi churna, Agnitundivati, Pippalyasav, Punarnava mandur, Navayas-
Dadam : Dadamadi churna, Lavanbhaskar churna.
Danti : Dantiyarista, Dantiyadi churna, Abhayarista, Chadraprutrharuti, Kishor guggal, visgarbha taila,
Devdar : Devdaryadi kwath, Devdaryadi churna, Devdarurasa, Sudarsan Churna, Punarnava mandur,
Dhamaso : Sudarsan churna, Haritakayadi kwath.
Dhana : Dhanyapanchak kwath, Gudchyadi kwath, Abhayarista, Lavanbhaskar churna.
Dhataki : Laghu gangadhar churna, Kutajarista, Abhayarista, Asokarist, khadirarista.
Dholimusli : Musli-pak, Musalyadi yog.
Dudhiovachnag : Kasisadi taila, Laghu vish garbh taila.
Eliachi (Ela) : Lavanbhaskar churna, Sitopaladi churna, Talidasichurna, Khadirarista, Chandraprabhavati.
Erand : Erand kwath, Rasna saptak kwath, Laghu vishgarbhtaila, Medicated erandoil.
Galo : Guduchyadi churna, Amristarista, Sudarsan churna, Guduchyadi kwath, Guduchi taila, Pippali
Gambhari garbhtaila. : Brihu-panchmooladi kwath, Kutujarista, Dasamularista.
Godhavaj : Saraswat churna, Pippalasav, Chandra prabha vati, Vachayog Sanjivanvati, Chandraprabha vati,
Gokhru : Dasmularishta, Gokshuroo-di kwath, Abhayarista, Gokshur guggal, Rasna Panchak kwath, Gokshuroo avleha, Haritakayadi kwath, Gokshuradi churna.
Guggal : Different types of guggal , Arogyavardini, Chandaprabhavati.
Gulab (Rosa) : Gulkand, Ark gulab, Talisadi churna, Sarpangadhayog.
Haldar : Laghu visgarbha taila, Pippaladiasava, Punarnavamandur, Sudarsan churna, Vidangadi lep.

Harde : Abhayarista, Agnitundivati, Sudarsan churna, Shringyadi churna, Arogyavardini, Chandraprabhavati,

Hing : Hingastak churna, Hingadivati rasonavati.

Indrajav : Amritarista, Laghu gangadhar churna, Punarnava mandur

Jaherkachoru : Laxmivilas rasa, Agni tundi vati, Sulhara-yog.

Jaifal : Sudarsan churna, Khadirarista.

Jamalgota : Jamalgotadi churna with chavedi, Naracha Rasa.

Jatamansi : Dashang lep, Laghu vishgarbh taila, Pippaliyasav.

Jethimadh : Sudharsan churna, Yastadi kwath, Tindu taila.

Jiru : Jirakayadiasi, Lavan bhaskar churna, Amiritarista, Agnitundi vati, Hingastak churna.

Jivanti : Sudarsan churna.

Kadu : Arogya vardhini, Sudarsan churna, Amritarista,

Kakadsingi : Shringyadi churna, Balchatur bhadra rasa.

Kalamari : Marichiadi ghrit, Marichiadi churna.

Kali jeeri : Somraj taila and Somraj grihta.

Kanchnar : Kanchnar guggal, Kanchanradi-vati.

Kankoi : Khadirarista, Chamdanadi-vati.

Kapilo : Krimigatini vati.

Kapur kachi : (Sati) Satyada churna, Satyadi kwath, Chandraprabhavati.

Kapur : Kapurasav, Amritanjan, Chandanadi vati, Vedantakrasa.

Karanj : Karanjadi churna, Karanjadi yog, Vidangadi lepa.

Karen : Laghu vish garbha taila.

Kariyatu : Sudarshan churna, Panch bhadra kwath, Chandraprabhavati.

Kaucha : Vanarigutika.

Khair : Khadirarista, Kutujarista, Lavangadi Vati, Khadiradi kwath, Khadiradi vati.

Kunwarpathu : Kumariasav, Kumarivati.

Kusta:(Kuth) : Laghu vishgarbh taila, Dasang lep, Pippalyasav.

Lasan : Rasonvati, Garlic capsules.

lauha, Yograj guggal, Vishgarbha-taila, Arogyavardhini, Chandraprabhavati.

Lavang (Loung)	:	Lavangadi churna, Pippalyasav, Lavangadi vati, Khadirarista, Sudarshan churna.
Lindi Peeper	:	Sudarsan choorna, Abhayarista, Punarnavamandur Pippalaysav, Yograj guggal, Chandraprabhavati.
Lodh	:	Lodhrasav, Pippalyasav.
Mahudo	:	Kutajarista, Pathyadi churna, Madhukasav.
Majith	:	Manjisthadi kwath, Karanjadi taila, Laghu vish garbh taila.
Malkangni	:	Jyotismati taila, Karanjadi yog, Laghu vish garbha taila.
Mocharasa	:	Laghu gangadhar choorna, Abhayarista.
		mooladikwath, Rasna saptak kwath, Yograj guggal, Kishorguggal.
Nagkesar	:	Amritarista, Lavan bhaskar churna, Khadirarista, Pipplayasav.
Nagod	:	Nirangundadi taila.
		Narayan taila.
Nasotar (Trivrit)	:	Abhayrista, Punarnava mandur, Kishor guggal.
		navayas loha, Pathyadi kwath and Pathyadi churna.
		Navayasloha, Sringadichurna, Visgarsha tel, Arogyavardhini, Khadirarista, Chandraprabhavati,
Parwal	:	Patoladi kwath, Sudarshan churna, Amrutadi Guggal.
Pasanbhed	:	Pasanvedadi kwath, Haritkayadi kwath.
Pippalimool	:	Pippalasav, Agnitundi vati, Chandraprabhavati, Pipalimuladi kwath, Goksuradi kwath,
Pittpapdo	:	Parpatyadiarista, Sudarshan churna, Panchbhadra kwath, Amritarista.
		Punarnava mandur, Navayasloha, Talisadi churna, Trikatu churna, Karanajadi yog, Hafketnrasa
		Punarnava mandur, Yograj guggal, Kutjaristu.
		Punarnava mandur.
		Punarnavamandur, Navayasiloha, Pippladi qwath, Shringyadi choorna, Karanjadi yog.
Pushkar mool	:	Pushkaradi churna, Sudarshan churna, Punarnava-mandur.
Rakta chandaṇ	:	Dashanglep, Parapatadi kwath, Guduchyadi kwath.
Rasna	:	Rasna saphtak kwath, Laghu vish garbh taila, Rasnadi gugal, Rasnadi kwath, Dashmoola kwath,
Rati satodi	:	Punarnavastak, Punarnavastak mandur, Punarnavastak vati, Punarnavastak kwath.
Sarasdo (siris)	:	Dasang lepa.
Sarpagandha	:	Sarpagandhadi churna, Sarpagandhadi yog, Sarpagandhadi vati.
Sarsav	:	Vidangsadi lep.

Satyanasini : Laghu vish garbh taila.

Shankhpushpi : Amrityadi rasayan.

Shatavari : Shatavari ghrita, Satamulyadi loha, Narayan taila, Vishnu taila.

Simlo : Shalmoli ghrita, Laghu gangadhar churna.

Sonamukhi : Panchaskar churna.

Sringadi churna, Talisadi churna.

Suva : Arkasona.

Taj (Dalchini) : Sitopaladi churna, Sudarshan churna, Lavanbhaskar churna, Talisadi churna.

Tal (Til) : Laghu vish garbh taila, Tiladi taila.

Talispatra : Talisadi vati and churna, Sudarshan churna, Lavanbhaskar churna.

Tetu : Dashmoola rista.

Vachanag : Mritunjivarasa, Agni tundi vati, Soubhagyvati, Sanjivani vati, Anand bhairav rasa, Laghu vish

Vad : Naygrodhadi churna.

Valiari : Sitopladi churna, Satpushpa arka, Abhayrista, Panchaskar churna.

Varuni : Abhiyarista, Narayan churna.

Vasadi kwath, Goksuradiguggal, Haritkadi kwath, Vidangadi lep, Khadirarista, Laghu vishgarbh taila,

Vidanga : Vidangyadi churna, Sudarshan churna, Vidanguvati, Agni tundi vati, Vidunagyadi arishta, Punarnava mandur, Guggal, Navayas loha, Vidangadi lepa, Kishor guggal, Chandraprabha vati.

Vidangadi loha.

Vidari : Chavyanprash.

Viroja chir (H) : Chandadivati.

Visgarbha taila, Khadirarista, Chandraprabhavati.

Chapter–6

SOME LESSER KNOWN MEDICINAL PLANTS

Adharamula	:	*Adenostemma lavenia* (L.) O. Kuntze. (Asteraceae). Lvs. (Stimulant, bruises, antiseptic).
Himamlika	:	*Antidesma acidum* Retz. (Euphorbiaceae). WP, Lvs, Frt. (Anasacra, Veneral disease, Dropsy).
Naganyavrnta	:	*Antirrhinum oronticum* Linn. (Scrophulariaceae). Frt and Lvs. (Epitaxis, enteric-fever).
Trikona bija	:	*Byttneria herbacea* Roxb. (Sterculiaceae). Rt and St. (Starch). (Bone fractures, sprains, menorrhagia, for sore in cattles- Veterinary practice).
Mukhapriya	:	*Erycibe paniculata* Roxb. (Convolvulaceae). Bk –In cholera, Syphilis, Lvs and st – useful in sprains of cattles.
Lohitapuspaka	:	*Hybanthus enneaspermus* (L.) F. Muell. (Ionidium enneaspermus (L.) Vent (Violaceae). Lvs-
Demulcent		and useful in hepatic diseases, Rts – Asthma, WP – Syphilis, impotency, Gonorrhoea.
Gojika	:	*Launaea nudicaulis* Hook. f. (Asteraceae). WP- galactogogue, Rt – constipation.
Nadibaya	:	*Myxopyrum serratulum* A. W. Hill (Oleaceae). Lvs – Respiratory tract infections, Rheumatoid arthritis, Neuralgia.

Chapter–7

AILMENTS VIS – A – VIS DIET

Disorders Vis-A-Vis Diet : Recommended (+VE), Contraindicated (-VE)

Stomach : (+ve) → wheat, bottlegourd, parval, milk, fresh curd. (-ve) → pulses, tea, narcotics, spicy articles, fried items and radish.

Intestial : (+ve) khichdi, green vegetables, buttermilk, banana, (-ve) → spicy masala, sugar, fried items.

Heart and Nervine : (+ve) cold and sweet preparations, curd, wheat, green vegetables. (-ve) → hot spicy food, beverages and fried items.

Respiratory : (+ve) wheat, dudhi, green vegetables, milk with pepper & Turmeric, (-ve) → rice, curd, pickles, fried articles.

Muscular : (+ve) milk, curd, green vegetables. (-ve) → heavy food, brinjal, rice, tea, fried articles.

Bone Joints : (+ve) banana, dates, milk. (-ve) → onion, potato, rice, fried preparations, tomatoes.

Blood : (+ve) wheat, cow's ghee, bottlegoud, bittergoud, karela, parval. (-ve) → rice, salt, radish, potato.

Urino-genital : (+ve) wheat, green vegetables, bottlegoud, cow's ghee. (-ve) → pulses, sweets, tomato, palak, excess of salt.

Plants Specific to Body Organs:

Mouth, Tooth and Gum : Tooth infection, pyorrohoea, toothache. (Bakul and Triphala, Kuth).

Eyes : Conjunctivitis, cataract, blindness (Chimed, Trifala Rasanajan).

Ears : Infections, deafness (Paribhadra, Anantmool, Neem, Nagod).

Hairs : Whitehairs, dandruff, alopeceia (Maka, Nagli, Katu Padval, Custurd Apple seeds, Neem).

Skin : Ringworm, eczema, leucoderma, soriasis, scabies, leprosy, vitiligo (Bavachi, Chakramard, Manjistha).

Brain : Tumor, depression, meningitis (Brahmi, Jatamansi, Ghodavach).

Nervous : Hemiplegia (Jyotismati, Kaucha, Brahmi).

Joints and Muscles : Inflammation, frozen shoulders, pain, rheumatism (Nagod, Rasna, Sunth, Erand, Guggal).

Heart and blood circulation : High and low BP, conjustion, burning, (Satodi, Arjun, Peepal leaves).

Lungs :	Tonsilitis, dyptheria, pharyngitis, TB, cancer, asthma (Ardusi, Bharangi, Kantkari ,Sirish & Mindhiaval).
Stomach, Liver and Spleen :	Oesophagitis, ulcers, anorexia, cirrhosis, spleenomegali, hyperacidity (Amla, Jethimadh, Sarpankho, Kalmegh, Shatavari Brahmi, Sarpankho, Aloevera, Amruta).
Intestine and Anus :	Heliminthiasis, diarrhoea, constipation, piles, colitis (Harde, Bili, Garmalo, Nagkesar, Kutaj, Vavding, Kampilak, Kuberaksh).
Genito-urinal Organs :	Renal stones, micturations, dysmenorrhoea, leucorrohea (Ashok, Lodhra, Gokhru, Vayvarno, Kalancho, Satodi).
Blood Purification and Virus :	(Galo, Sariva, Khair, Kariyatu, Manjistha).
Endocrinal glands :	Thyroid related symptoms (Kanchnar). Pancreas related symptoms (Medhasingi).
Tonic (Energy) :	For vitality (Amla, Galo, Brahmi, Aswagandha, Satavari, Bala, Kaucha, Shankhpushpi).

Chapter–8

MEDICINAL PLANTS AND THEIR PROPERTIES

LATIN NAME AND FAMILY	NAMES (S, G, M, H, E).	PARTS USED	MEDICINAL PROPERTIES USES/ APPLICATIONS/ACTIVITIES	REMARKS/SPECIFIC ACTIVITIES/ SIDE EFFECTS IF ANY
Abelmoschus moschatus (L.) Medik. (Malvaceae)	Latakasturika-katuk (S), Kasturibhindo (G). Musk Mallow, Ambrette (E).	Seeds	Useful in nervous debility, asthma, hysteria and convulsions, stomachic disorders. Helitotis.	Seeds Chewed, oil in perfumery.
Abrus precatorius Linn. (Fabaceae)	Gunja (S), Chanothi (G), Rati (H), Gunj (M). Bead Plant / Crab's Eye, (E) Indian Liquorice, Rosary Pea	Roots, Leaves, seeds.	Hair tonic, laxative, antiphlogistic, aphrodisiac.	Dried root is used as a substitute to Glycyrrhiza. Seeds coat posinous, Kerwells useful.
Abutilon indicum Sweet. (Malvaceae)	Atibala (S), Kanski (G), Kandhi (H), Mudra (M). Country Mallow (E).	Roots, Leaves, Seeds.	Demulcent, aphrodisiac, laxative, diuretic, sedative. Useful in fever, gonorrhoea, renal stones, leprosy, haemorrhoids and inflammation of the bladder & gums.	It is an anti-oxidant.
Acacia chundra Willd. (Mimosaceae)	Khadir (S), Khair (G),Catechu Tree (E).	Bark, Seed. Gum , wood extract	Aphrodisiac, antidote to poisoning, astringent, expectorant, bronchial affections, cancer, chronic ulceration, diarrhoea, dysentery, epistaxis, haemoptyxis, haemorrhage, ulcers, biles and eruptions of the skin.	Agglutenins from seeds used in leukemia.
Acacia leucophloea (Roxb.) Willd. (Mimosaceae)	Irimed (S), Ambiyar (G), Panthribabul (M), Safed babul (H).	Bark	Astringent, pyorrhea, antiseptic.	Stops Tooth ache.

S =Sanskrit, G =Gujrat, M =Marathi, H =Hindi, E =English

Acacia nilotica (L.) Del subsp. *indica* (Bth.) Brenan. (Mimosaceae)	Babul (S), Deshibaval (G), Babul (H, M). Babul Tree (E).	Bark, Gum Fruit	Anthelmintic, antidote, aphrodisiac, astringent, demulcent, diuretic, emollient, expectorant, nutritive, soothing, dysentery, diarrhoea, leucorrhoea, leprosy and piles.	"EKAKIA" is the Arabic name given to preparation made from dried fruits.
Acalypha indica Linn.(Euphorbiaceae)	Haritamanjari (S), Kupi (G), Indian Acalypha (E).	Whole plant	Anthelmintic, scabies, rheumatoid arthritis, bronchitis, asthma, earaches, syphilitic ulcers and in acute mania, skin affections.	----
Achyranthes aspera L. (Amaranthaceae)	Apamarga (S), Aghedo (G), Aghada (M), Chirchita (H).Chaff Tree, Rough Chaff (E).	Root, Leaves, Seed, Whole Plant.	Used in curing diuretic affections in renal dropsies, stomachache, bowel complaints, piles, boil and skin eruptions, binge eating disorders, toothache.	In large doses produces abortion inducing labour pains. Chemoprotective activity reported.
Aconitum ferox (Bruhl.) Muk. (Ranunculaceae)	Vatsanabh (S), Vachnag (G), Bachnag (H), Kalavachnag (M). Munk's Hood (E)	Root	Alterative, antiarthritic, debility, diaphoretic, diuretic, expectorant, febrifuge, narcotic, nervine tonic and Stomachic. Indicated in asthma, diabetes, dyspepsia, leprosy, paralysis, rheumatism, spermatorrhoea and typhoid.	Contraindicated in patients with hyperacidity, T. B. and impotency. Its antidote is Tandaljo, Hardar, Tea, Coffee, and Whisky. Injections of cardiac glycosides especially of Digitalis purpurea Digoxin.
Aconitum heterophyllum Wall.(Ranunculaceae)	Ativisha (S), Ativis (G).	Tuberous Roots.	Stomachic, aphrodisiac, tonic, antiperiodic, astringent, anthelmintic.	----
Acorus calamus Linn.(Araceae)	Ugra-gandha (S), Vekhand (M), Vachh (G, H).	Dried rhizomes.	Dry piles, hysteria, eczema, scabies and acidity, Nervinetonic.	Highly useful in dysentery, bronchial coughing and asthma.
Adhatoda zeylanica Medic. (Acanthaceae)*Justicia adhatoda*	Vasa (S), Ardusi (G), Adusa (M), Vasa (H).Vasaka (E).	Root, Leaves, Whole Plant.	Alterative, analgesic, anti-arthritic, antiseptic, anti-spasmodic, diuretic, expectorant, febrifuge, laxative, neuralgic and sedative. Used in curing asthma, chronic bronchitis, chest complaints, haeomptysis, leprosy, pulmonary affections, scabies and skin diseases.	Gingival inflammation and Pyorrhoea. Contraindicated in pregnancy.
Aegle marmelos Linn. (Rutaceae)	Bilva (S), Bila (G), Bailphal (M), Bel (H).Bael fruit, stone apple, bengal quince (E).	Root pulp, roots.	Alterative, antipyretic, antiscorbutic, astringent, digestive, febrifuge, laxative, nutritive, stimulant, stomachic and tonic. Best Anti-Diarrhoel, Anti-Dysentric, Coolant.	Antifungal and anti-ulcer activity reported.

Aerva lanata (L.) Juss. (Amaranthaceae)	Bhadrika (S), Gorakhganja (G).	Root, Seeds	Demulcent and tonic. Used in headache, gonorrhoea, kidney disorders, cutaneous affections and sugar in urine, seeds diaretic.	——-
Alangium salvifolium (L. f.) Wang. (Alangiaceae)	Ankollak (S), Ankol (G, M, H).	Root, Leaves, Fruit.	Laxative, blood purifier, antidote, febrifuge, cooling and nutritive.	Makes manure, Fruit pulpedible.
Albizia lebbeck (L.) Willd. (Mimosaceae)	Siris (S, G), Black Sirash (M), Siras (H).	Whole plant	Aphrodisiac, astringent, collyrium, expectorant, tonic. Useful in asthma, enlargement of cervical gland, diarrhoea, night blindness, piles and scrofula.	Healing wounds, syphilis and seed oil is highly effective in leprosy. Local inflammatory reactions in throat and vagina are the major side effects.
Alhagi psuedalhagi (M. Bieb.) Deav.(Fabaceae)	Gandhari (S), Dhamaso (G), Javas (H, M).Camel's Thorn (E).	Root and whole plant	Laxative, diuretic, expectorant and cholagogue.	——-
Allium sativum Linn.(Liliaceae)	Ugra-gandha (S), Lasan (G), Garlic (E).	Bulbs.	Alterative, antiarthritic, cholagogue, digestive, emmenagogue, expectorant, febrifuge, rubefacient, stimulant, tonic and vermifuge. Used in cough, facial palsy, fatigue, flatulence, fever, hysteria, leprosy, piles, rheumatism, sciatica, swelling and worms.	In large doses may cause sorethroat. Aggravates piles.
Aloe indica Linn.(Liliaceae)	Kumari (S), Kunvarpathu (G), Korpath (M), Gwar path (H), Indian Aloes (E).	Leaves. Mucilage/ juice from the leaves.	Laxative, emmenagogue, alterative, blood purifier, abortifacient, anthelmintic, tonic, cooling, carminative, cathartic, purgative and stomachic. Useful in amenorrhoea, dyspepsia, glandular enlargement and spleen disorders, jaundice, menstrual suppressions, rectal fissure.	Contraindicated in pregnancy, lactation, kidney complaints and irritated bowel complaints. Immuno-modulatory and radio protective efficacy reported. Analgesic, anti-inflammatory.
Alstonia scholaris (Linn.) R. Br. (Apocynaceae)	Sapta-parna (S), Saptaparni (G) Satvin (M, H). Devil's Tree (E).	Bark, Leaves.	Increases lactation, useful in cough, asthma and idiopathic psoriasis. Bark antimalarial.	——-

Amorphophalus campanulatus (Schott.) Engler.(Araceae)	Kand-nayak (S), Ghodasuren (M), Suran (G, H), Elephant's Foot Yam (E).	Corm.	Useful in culinary purposes, piles, restorative in dyspepsia, debility and boils.	——-
Andrographis paniculata (Burm. f.) Wall. (Acanthaceae)	Kalpatha (S), Kalmegh (G) Alekirayat (M), Lilu-karyata (H).	Dried aerial parts.	Alterative, anthelmintic, febrifuge, stomachic and tonic.	Immunostimulant, appetizer. Side effects- vomiting.
Anethum graveolens Linn. (Apiaceae)	Sat-pushpa (S), Suwa (G), Balantshep (M), Soya (H), Dill Seeds (E).	Seed.	Anthelmintic, cardiac, carminative, diaphoretic, diuretic, emmenagogue, expectorant, febrifuge, stomachic. Useful in curing seminal weakness, asthma, fever, skin diseases and vomiting.	Galactagogue, good for lactating mother.
Anogeissus latifolia Guill. (Combretaceae)	Pisachvruksha (S), Dhavdo (G), Dhavada (M), Dhava (H).	Wood, Bark, gum	Demulcent, hay-asthma and astringent. Gum edible, laxative.	——-
Argemone mexicana Linn. (Papaveraceae)	Swarnakshiri (S), Satyanasi (H), Darudi (G Mexican Poppy (E).	Root and Seed oil	Alterative, aperient, demulcent, emetic, expectorant, laxative, suppurative and narcotic. Useful in cutaneous affections, conjunctivitis, dropsy, dysentery, leprosy and ulcers.	Mostly adulterated with mustard oil for profiteering. Causes ascitis- dropsy.
Argyreia nervosa (Burm. f.) Boj. (Convolvulaceae)	Samudraphalaka (S), Samudrasosh, Vardharo (G), Samudrà shoku (M), Bidhara (H), Elephant Creeper wooly Asia Glory.(E).	Roots, seeds and leaves	Cures synovitis and syphilis. Used as nervine tonic and revitalizes the body; boils, skin affections.	Increases suppuration.
Aristolochia bracteolata Lam.(Aristolochiaceae)	Nakuli (S), Gandhan (M), Kidamari (G),Birtter Wort (E).	Leaves, stem, roots.	Purgative, emmenagogue, alterative, antiperiodic and anthelmintic. Useful in amenorrhoea, dysmenorrhoea, intermittent fever, syphilis, gonorrhoea and skin diseases.	Leaf juice with Castor Oil very effective in psora.
Asparagus racemosus Willd var. *javanicus* Baker. (Liliaceae)	Bahu-putra (S)Satavari (G), Wild Asparagus (E).	Roots	Anti-diarrhoeal, antidysenteric, antispasmodic, aphrodisiac, cardiac tonic, general tonic, carminative, demulcent, diuretic, galactagogue, nervine tonic.	Anti-oxidant. Specific dose-5-10 grains.

Azadirachta indica Juss. (Meliaceae)	Nimb (S), Limbdo (G), Kadunimb (M), Nimb (H), Neem Plant, Margosa Tree (E).	Stem bark, leaves, root bark.	Anthelmintic, antimalarial, antiperiodic, antiseptic, appetizer, astringent, bitter tonic, constipative, contraceptive (oral), demulcent, emmenagogue, emollient, expectorant, febrifuge, purgative, stimulant, stomachic and vermifuge. Useful in digestion, catarrhal affections, diabetes, debility, eczema, erysipelas, fever, jaundice, leprosy, liver complaints, lumbago, prurigo, rheumatism, scrofula, ulcers, urticaria, vomiting in fever.	Azadirachtin is an Anti-Bavterial, Anti-Fungal, Anti-Viral, Oil Cake make manure Pest repelient, Anti-Feedent.
Bacopa monnieri (L.) Pennell. (Scrophulariaceae)	Tiktalonika (S), Newari (G), Brahmi (H), Indian Penny Wort (E).	Dried Whole Plant.	Aperient, aphrodisiac, diuretic, laxative, nervine tonic, bronchitis, insanity, dropsy, jaundice, epilepsy and hysteria.	Anti-epileptic, anti-oxidant, anti-ulcer, spasmolytic.
Balanites aegyptiaca (Linn.) Delile.(Balanitaceae)	Tailaphala (S), Ingori (G).	Seeds, Bark, Flowers, Leaves.	Aphrodisiac, anthelmintic, carminative, diuretic, expectorant, purgative and vermifuge. Useful in asthma, blood eruptions, cough and colic, constipation and skin diseases.	----
Baliospermum montanum (Willd.) Muell. Euphorbiaceae)	Danti (S), Danti (G, M, H).	Roots, seeds.	Drastic purgative, anaemia and piles.	For laxative effect, one to two grain with trikatu is advised.
Barleria prionitis Linn. (Acanthaceae)	Karunta (S), Kantaserio (G).	Leaves, Roots.	Used in catarrhal affections, glandular swellings, boils, whooping cough and dropsy.	----
Bauhinia purpurea Linn. (Caesalpiniaceae)	Asmantak (S), Asitro (G), Apto (M), Sirhata (H).	Root bark, seeds, fruits.	Antidote to poisons. Useful in curing biliousness, purifies blood, venereal diseases, bladder stone, leprosy, swellings and asthma.	----
Bauhinia variegata L.(Caesalpiniaceae)	Yamalpatrak (S), Asotaro (G), Kanchnar Kavidara (M), Kovidar (H).	Root bark, leaves, fruits.	Alterative, anthelmintic, anti-rheumatic, astringent, expectorant, tonic. Cures diarrhoea, dyspepsia, internal worms, leprosy, menorrhagia, piles and scrofula Tumors.	Good on Liver Disfunction.

Berberis aristata Roxb. ex DC.(Berberidaceae)	Daruharidra (S), Daruhaldi (H), Indian Barberry (E).	Root, stem bark	Alterative, antiperiodic, antipyretic, bitter tonic, diaphoretic, ophthalmic, and styptic. Useful in bilious symptoms, diarrhoea, conjunctivitis, febrifuge, hepatitis, inflammatory swellings, jaundice, malarial dyspepsia, menorrhagia, neuralgia, remittent fever and ulceration.	----
Boerhavia diffusa Linn.(Nyctaginaceae)	Punarnava (S),Satodi (G),Punarnava (H). Spreading Hog Weed (E).	Whole Plant	Aphrodisiac, cardiac stimulant, diaphoretic, diuretic, dropsy, emetic, expectorant. Used in internal inflammation, febrifuge, laxative, leucorrhoea, jaundice, asthma, and constipation.	Causes vomiting. Immuno-modulatory activity reported.
Bombax ceiba Linn.(Bombacaceae)	Mocha (S), Shimdo (G), Shanvar (M), Silk Cotton Tree (E). Ratishalmali.	Gum, soft root, lowers, seeds prickle.	Useful in curing intestinal disorders, emetic, convulsive fits, menorrhagia, weakness of the genital organs, pimples.	----
Boswellia serrata Roxb. ex Colebr.(Burseraceae)	Sallaki (S), Saladi (G), Sallai vruksh (M). Indian Sallaki (E).	Gum	Used in curing cough and cold, purifies blood, dysentery, rheumatism, skin diseases, ulcers, antidote to snake bites and scorpion sting.	Good on Liver Dysfunction, Vatroga.
Buchanania lanzan Spreng. (Anacardiaceae)	Piyalaka (S), Charoli (G), Chironji (M, H)	Fruit, seeds.	Sweet and laxative. Nutritious and tonic, Galactogogue.	Seeds nutritive used as a dry fruit.
Butea monosperma (Lamk.) Taub.(Fabaceae)	Palasa (S), Khakhro (G), Dhak (M), Palash (H), Flame of the Forest (E).	Seed, gum. Flowers, leaves	Aperient, rubefacient, astringent, aphrodisiac. Useful in boils and pimples, flatulence and colic, promotes menstrual flow, diuretic, purgative, sunstroke.	----
Caesalpinia crista Linn. (Caesalpiniaceae)	Putikaranj (S), Kanchka (G), Sagargota (M), Kanta-karanj (H).	Root bark, kernel leaves, seed oil.	Cures fever, colic, asthma, hydrocele and glandular swellings, convulsion, paralysis, nervous complaints and liver complaints, anthelmintic.	Post natal care and fever (Novel activities).

Callophyllum inophyllum Linn.(Clusiaceae)	Punga (S), Undi (G, M), Sultana champa (H).	Root bark, seed wax tincture of leaves	Indicated in rheumatism and scabies. Also useful in syphilis, eczema, insanity and internal haemorrhages. Tincture of leaves highly useful in cold, cough, fever and asthma.	Seed wax may provide good material for cosmetics.
Calotropis procera (Aiton.) R. Br.(Asclepiadaceae)	Ark (S), Akando (G), Rui (M), Aak (H).	Whole Plant except stem.	Alterative, anodyne, antiperiodic, antispasmodic, blood purifier, cardiac, diaphoretic, digestive, emetic, expectorant, sedative, stomachic and suppurative, anti-malarial.	——-
Cardiospermum helicacabum Linn.(Sapindaceae)	Karnasphota (S), Kagdolio (G), Kanphuti (M), Nayphatki (H), Winter cherry, Balloon vine (E).	Root, leaves, whole plant.	Vitilego, anti-inflammatory, given to promote catamenial flow during menstrual period, rheumatism, nervous disorders, chronic bronchitis, amenorrhoea, bilious affections, sore eyes, hernia.	Leaves highly useful in chronic rheumatoid arthritis, whereas in early pains of joints root decoction is used.
Careya arborea Roxb. (Lecythidaceae)	Kumbhi (S, G, H), Kumbia (M).	Roots and bark.	Heals ruptures after childbirth, antidote to snake bite and ulcers.	Seeds poisonous if consumed.
Cassia absus Linn.(Caesalpiniaceae)	Vanya-kulath (S), Chimed (G), Chinol (M), Chaksu (H).	Seeds.	Highly effective in blood purification and mucus disorders.	Anti-Conjunctivitis.
Cassia angustifolia Linn.(Caesalpiniaceae)	Markandi (S), Sonamukhi Mindhiawal (G). Indian Senna (E).	Dried leaves	Anthelmintic, attenuant, blood purifier, cathartic, purgative. Useful in bile troubles, constipation, haemorroids, gout and rheumatism, fistula in ano.	Exclusively cultivated in Kachchh.
Cassia fistula Linn.(Caesalpiniaceae)	Rajavriksha (S), Garmalo (G), Bahwa (M), Amaltas (H), Indian Laburnum (E).	Fruits.	Emetic, febrifuge, laxative, lenitive, purgative. Cures dyspepsia, constipation, indigestion, fever and cardiac diseases.	Skin diseases and lymph inflammations.
Cassia occidentalis L. (Caesalpiniaceae)	Kasari (S), Kasundro (G), Kasvida (M), Kasondi (H), Negrocoffee (E)	Roots, leaves, seeds.	Potential remedy in hysteria and spasms. Tumours.	Anti-oxidant. Seeds Roasted, powdered, boiled and drunk as coffee.

Cassia tora Linn. (Caesalpiniaceae)	Chakramarda (S), Kunvadio (G), Takala (M), Chakvad (H).Ring Worm Plant (E)	Leaves, seeds.	Aperient, antiparasitic, germicidal, suppurative. Cures skin diseases especially eczema, leprosy, psoriasis, tumour and ulcers.	Anti-oxidant. Seeds are used in French coffee.
Catharanthus roseus (Linn.) G. Don.(Apocynaceae)	Suhagan (S), Barmasi (G), Sadaphul (M), Sadabahar (H), Periwrinkle (E)	Roots, Whole Plant.	Most potential anti-cancerous drug. Anti-diabetic, cures hypotension.	——-
Celastrus paniculata Willd.(Celastraceae)	Jyotishmati (S), Malkangni (G), Malkakna (M, H).	Fruits and Seeds.	Anodyne, aphrodisiac, brain tonic, carminative, diaphoretic, diuretic, emmenagogue, expectorant, febrifuge, nervine tonic, stimulant. Cures asthma, beriberi, colic, constipation, fever, loss of memory, paralysis and scrofula.	Anti-radical and DNA cleavage protectors. Cyto-toxic.
Celosia argentea Linn. (Amaranthaceae)	Srivalliika (S), lampdi (G), Sarvali (M, H)	Seed, Whole Plant.	Lithiotriptic, sedative and diuresis.	——-
Centella asiatica (Linn.) Urb. (Apiaceae)	Mandukparni (S), Brahmi (G, M, H).	Whole plant.	Nervine tonic, blood purifier, increases memory, cures anxiety neurosis, sedative and alterative.	Caution- contact dermatitis. Possible carcinogenic with repeated uses.
Chlorophytum borivilianum Sant. and Fernand. (Liliaceae)	Svet musli (S)Safedmusli (G), Musali (M, H).	Roots.	Aphrodisiac, oligospermia, anorexia, piles, tuberculosis, anaemia, impotency, galactagogue, analgesic (Muscular pain) and leucorrhoea.	——-
Cinchona calisaya (Rubiaceae).	Cinchona (G, M, H).	Dried bark	Most potent medicine for malarial fever. Local application in rheumatism.	In high doses cause nausea and deafness. Contraind-icated in pregnancy, cardiac patients.
Cissampelos pareira Linn. (Menispermaceae)	Laghupatha (S), Karandhiyu (G), Path (H), Padavel (M).	Root and Leaves	Piles and as tonic, diuretic, astringent, sedative, genito-urinary troubles, cough and heart complaints.	——-

Cissus quadrangularis Linn.(Vitaceae)	Asthi-samhar (S), Hadsankad (G), Hadjod (H), Kandvel (M).	Leaves and twigs.	Alterative, stimulant, astringent, dislocations, sores, fractured limbs.	Anti-inflammatory and neuroprotective (New activity reported).
Citrullus colocynthis (Linn.) Schrad.(Cucurbitaceae)	Indravaruni (S), Kadvabhotingda (G), Indrayan (M, H). Bitter Apple (E).	Roots, fruits.	Aboritifacient, acrid, appetizer, blood purifier, cathartic, drastic purgative, febrifuge, biliousness, jaundice, cerebral congestion, constipation and fever.	Rheumatoid arthritis and splenomegaly. Should be used in combination with other drugs and not as single drug. Side effects- intestinal inflammation in large doses.
Clerodendrum multiflorum Baker.(Verbenaceae)	Agnimanth (S), Arni (G), Ganiyari (H), Airan-takli (M).	Root and leaves.	Alterative, astringent, useful in cervical adenitis, anti-obesity.	Leaves used as Spinach.
Clerodendrum serratum (L. f.) Gaertn. (Verbenaceae)	Bharangi (S), Bhargi, Bhabhneta (H), Bharang (G, M).	Root, bark, leaves	Anthelmintic, carminative, diaphoretic, digestive, expectorant, febrifuge and suppurative. Useful in asthma, catarrhal affections, cephalic and ophthalmic, dropsy, scrofula.	——-
Clitorea ternatea Linn. (Fabaceae)	Aparajita (S), Kaligai (G), Butterfly Pea (E).	Leaves Root	Demulcent, diuretic, laxative, hemicrania, cervical adenitis., Oligospermia.	——-
Cocculus hirsutus (Linn.) Diels. (Menispermaceae)	Patalgarudi (S), Vevadi (G), Jaljamni (H), Tan (M).	Roots and leaves	Highly useful in rheumatism, acute gonorrhoea, acidity, blood purifier.	It chould be used as substitute for Tinospora sp and Hemidesmus. sp.
Commiphora wightii (Arnott.) Bhandari.(Burseraceae)	Devdhupa (S), Guggal (G, M, H)). Indian Bedellium (E).	Oleo-gum-resin	Alterative, demulcent, stimulant, tonic, antispasmodic, emmenagogue, anti-rheumatic, cures anxiety neurosis, scrofulous affections.	Hypolipidaemic. Contraindicated in pregnancy. Side effects- skin rash and diarrhoea.

Convolvulus microphyllus (Roth) Sieb. ex Spr. (Convolvulaceae)	Shankhavali (S), Shankhpushpi (G, H), Shankhaveli (M).	Whole plant.	Alterative, antiphlegmatic, antiphlogistic, anthelmintic, cephalic. Cures dysentery, insomnia, stomachic, nervine tonic. Effective in high blood pressure.	Anti-oxidant.
Coptis treeta Wall.(Ranunculaceae)	Mamirah (S), Pitmula (H), Haldiya bachnag (M).	Dried rhizomes	Antidiabetic, bitter tonic, carminative, expectorant, febrifuge, ophthalmic, stomachic. Useful in nervous diseases, atonic dyspepsia, asthma and cough, jaundice, flatulence and visceral obstruction.	----
Cordia dichotoma Forst. f. (Ehretiaceae)	Bahuvarkara (S), Gunda (G), Bhonkar (M), Lasuda (H).	Fruit rind, Bark leaves.	Stomachache, rheumatism, asthma, antidote to poison, leprosy and ulcers, coughs, cardiac diseases and uterine diseases.	Psychic disturbances. Can be used for blackening hairs.
Crateva magna (Lour.) DC. (Capparaceae)	Varun (S), Vay-varno (G), Three leaved caper (E).	Root bark and leaves	Renal stone, tubercular gland and enlargement of liver.	Anti-lithiatic property reported.
Cuminum cyminum Linn. (Apiaceae)	Jiraka (S), Jiru (G), Jire (M), Jira (H), Cumin Seed (E).	Seed.	Anthelmintic, astringent, carminative, cooling, digestive, diuretic, febrifuge, stimulant, stomachic and tonic.	----
Curculigo orchioides Gaertn. (Hypoxidaceae)	Tala-patri (S), Kalimusli (G, H, M)..	Tubers.	Gonorrhoea, piles, debility, impotence and asthma, jaundice, diarrhoea and colic, scalds and blisters on skin, diabetes, hemorrhage, urino-genital disorders.	----
Curcuma longa Linn.(Scitaminaceae)	Haridra (S), Hardar (G), Hadad (M), Haldi (H), Turmeric (E).	Rhizome.	Alterative, anthelmintic, antiperiodic, antiparasitic, aromatic and astringent, bitter, carminative, hot, stimulant and tonic. Useful in boils, bruises, chronic bronchitis, cold, cough, coryza, eosinophilia, jaundice, swellings and skin diseases.	Anti-inflammatory and neuro-protective.

Cymbopogon martinii (Roxb.) Wats. (Poaceae)	Saugandhika (S), Rosaghass (G), Lemon Grass (E).	Leaves	Rheumatism, goiter and swellings of joints.	——-
Cyperus rotundus (L.) Pers.(Cyperaceae)	Mustaka (S), Nagarmoth Chido (G), Moth (M), Motha (H). Nut Grass (E).	Roots.	Anthelmintic, astringent, attenuant, carminative, demulcent, diaphoretic, diuretic, emmenagogue, expectorant, febrifuge, galactagogue, lithotriptic, nervine tonic, sedative, stomachic and tonic.	——-
Datura metel Linn.(Solanaceae)	Dhustur (S), Dhanturo (G)Dhatura (M, H), Thorn Apple (E).	Dried Leaves, flowers, Seeds.	Narcotic, anodyne, antiseptic, demulcent, digestive, antispasmodic, emetic, expectorant, intoxicating, sedative. Notable activity-anthelmintic. Toxicity consideration is required before using the plant.	Flowers hasten fermentation; added in preparing ayurvedic drugs. Side effects- dry ing of mouth and blurring of vision.
Desmodium gangeticum (Linn.) DC. (Fabaceae)	Saliparni (S), Salvan (G), Ranbhul (M), Sarivan (H).	Whole plant.	Tonic, promotes digestion, roots highly effective in rheumatic fever.	One of the ingredients of dasamularisht.
Desmostachya bipinnata (Linn.) Stapf. (Poaceae)	Yagna-bhusan (S), Dabh (G), Darbhu (M), Kans (H).	Roots	Astringent, diuretic, expectorant and stomachic. Diarrhoea, dysentery, leucorrhoea, menorrhagia, skin diseases and kidney stones.	——-
Dioscorea bulbifera Linn. (Dioscoreaceae)	Krodkunda (S)Dukarkand (G)Kadukrand (M), Varahikand (H)	Rhizome	Indicated as tonic, rheumatoid arthritis.	One of the ingredients of Chyavanprasha.
Diospyros melanoxylon Roxb.(Ebenaceae)	Tinduka (S), Timru (G), Taindu (M, H). Riberebany (E).	Bark, fruit, flower.	Indicated in boils, tumours, bilious fever, leprosy, gonorrhoea, blood diseases, asthma, chronic dysentery, diarrhoea, haemorrhages.	Fruits edible, sweet, and nutritive. Wood heavy, black, hard.
Dolichos biflorus Linn. (Fabaceae)	Kulatha (S), Kalthi (G), Lal-kulthi (M), Kulthi (H) Horse Gram (E).	Fruits.	Anthelmintic, antilithiatic, astringent, diaphoretic, diuretic, emmenagogue, expectorants, febrifuge and tonic. Used in asthma, hiccough, leucorrhoea, menstrual disorders, piles and worms, diaretic.	Tonic (New activity).

Eclipta alba (Linn.) Hassak. (Asteraceae)	Bhringraja (S), Safed bhangaro (G), Maka (M), Bhangra (H),Trailing Eclipta (E).	Whole Plant.	Tonic, alterative, emetic, purgative, anti-hepatic.	Anti-viral, broncho-dilator.
Elephantopus scaber Linn. (Asteraceae)	Gojihva (S), Hastipata (G), Pathri (M), Gobhi (H).	Roots Leaves.	Astringent, alterative, febrifuge, urinary sedative. Highly effective against hypoprothrombinaemia.	Antitumour.
Embelia tsjeriam-cottam (R. and S.) DC.(Myrsinaceae)	Chitratandoola (S), Vavding (G, M), Vay-vidang (H).	Ripe Fruits.	Antidote to snake venom, insanity, analgesic, anthelmintic, jaundice, anti-ageing.	Highly effective against tapeworms. Side effects-sexual debility. Potential oral contraceptive.
Enicostema littorale (Willd.) Verdcourt.(Gentianaceae)	Nagajihva (S), Mamejavo (G).	Leaves.	Blood purifier, dropsy, rheumatism, ulcers, hernia and swellings, anti-malarial.	——-
Ephedra gerardiana Wall. (Ephedraceae)	Soma (S, M, H, G), Ephedra (E).	Dried young stem.	Indicated in asthma, rheumatism, cardiac diseases, urinary disorders, and inflammation of mucous membrane, sinusitis, chronic asthmatic attacks, pneumonia, and diptheria.	Large doses be avoided leads to nausea, sweating and skin ailments.
Eulophia dabia (Don.) Hochr. (Orchidaceae)	Mucchhatak (S), Salam (H), Salempak (G), Salep (E).	Tubers/ rhizomes	Highly effective in piles and scanty urine. Oligospermia, azoospermia. Nutritive yet does not cause constipation. Tonic.	2 types- Panja salam and Lahasunia salam (Mishri)available. Dose-3 g.
Euphorbia hirta Linn.(Euphorbiaceae)	Dugdhika (S), Dudheli (G), Motidudhi (M), Badidudhi (H)Euphorbia (E).	Whole Plant, Leaves.	Indicated in ringworm, bleeding piles and highly effective in asthma.	Cardiac asthma and trachycardia.
Ferula asafoetida Regel. (Apiaceae)	Hingu (S), Hing (G, M, H), Asafoetida (E).	Root gum.	Useful in cough, gastritis, jaundice, rheumatism and repeated threatened abortion.	——-

Ficus benghalensis Linn. (Moraceae)	Vat (S), Vad (G), Bad (H). Banyan Tree (E).	Aerial roots, bark, fruits.	Anodyne, anti-arthritic, astringent, conceptive, cooling, diuretic, suppurative and tonic, diabetes, diarrhoea, dysentery, leucorrhoea, lumbago and tonic.	----
Ficus glomerata Linn.(Moraceae)	Audumbar (S), Umero (G), Goolar (H), Umbar (M).	Dried Bark, Leaves, unripe Fruits.	Astringent, carminative, stomachic, styptic, healing of wounds (antiseptic), alterative, tonic.	To protect from threatened abortion. Anti-inflammatory.
Ficus hispida Linn.(Moraceae)	Kakodumbar (S), Dhedumro (G), Kathgular (H), BoKhada (M).	Dried bark, leaves, unripe fruits, latex	Emetic and laxative, promote the secretion of milk and are supposed to preserve the foetus in the womb, leucoderma.	Latex causes blisters on skin.
Ficus religiosa Linn.(Moraceae)	Aswath (S), Pipalo (G), Sacred Fig (E).	Leaves, unripe fruits.	Alterative, aphrodisiac, astringent, cooling, expectorant, laxative, asthma, colic, constipation, diarrhoea and dysentery.	----
Foeniculum vulgare Mill. (Apiaceae)	Madhurika (S), Valyari (G), Badi shep (M), Badi shop (H), Fennel (E).	Seed.	Appetizer, cardiac stimulant, carminative, diaphoretic, diuretic, emmenagogue, expectorant, febrifuge, stomachic, stimulant, tonic, vermifuge and purgative.	----
Garcinia morella Roxb. (Clusiaceae)	Kankushta (S), Ravanchi (G).	Gum	Aperient, carminative, cardiac, diuretic, expectorant, emollient and stomachic.	Liver enlargement.
Gloriosa superba Linn. (Liliaceae)	Agnisikha (S), Dudhiovachhnag (G), Kalihari (H), Kandyanag (M), Malabar Glory Lily (E).	Roots.	Abortifacient, alterative, anthelmintic, antiperiodic, purgative, stimulant and tonic. Cures abscess, bile troubles, boils, leprosy, expels skin parasites and intestinal worms.	Poisonous.

Ipomoea sepiaria Koen. ex Roxb. (Convolvulaceae)	Lakshmana (S), Hanumanvel (G).	Roots, seeds.	Aphrodisiac and lactagogue. Controls menstrual discharges, tuberculosis, spleen and liver enlargement.	----
Jasminum arborescens Roxb. (Oleaceae)	Jati (S), Chameli (G, H, M), Spanish Jasmine (E).	Leaves, flowers	Aphrodisiac, anthelmintic, diuretic, emmenagogue, emollient, suppurative, impotency, headache, skin diseases, ulcers.	----
Jasminum multiflorum Andr. (Oleaceae)	Mallika (S), Mogro (G), Mogra (M), Motia (H).	Roots and flowers	Emetic, ringworms, herpes, bronchial asthma, phlegm, ophthalmic diseases.	----
Jatropha curcas (Euphorbiaceae)	Nayogradhi (S), Ratanjyot (G), Thordanti (M), Muglai errand (H).	Leaf juice, root, seed oil.	Laxative; increases milk flow, rheumatism, leprosy and haemorrhage.	Seeds yield oil equitable to diesel.
Lawsonia inermis Linn. (Lythraceae)	Madyantika (S), Deshimehndi (G), Heena Plant (E).	Fresh & powder-ed leaves.	Alterative, astringent, prophylactic against skin diseases, refrigerant, blood dysentery, boils, burns, calculous affection, enlargement of spleen, insomnia, jaundice, skin diseases and spermatorrhoea.	----
Lepidium sativum Linn. (Brassicaceae)	Chandrasur (S), Halim (H), Ashelio (G)	Seeds	Useful in seminal debility, leucorrhoea, rheumatism, lumbago, hiccup, diarrhoea, as blood purifier and chronic enlargement of spleen, galactagogue.	Seeds used along with milk internally cause abortion. Not to be given during pregnancy, best post partum.

Glycyrrhiza glabra Linn. (Fabaceae)	Yastimadhu (S), Jethimadh (G, M), Mulethi (H), Indian Liquorice (E).	Roots and stolons.	Cooling, demulcent, diuretic, emmenagogue, emollient, febrifuge, laxative, ophthalmic, restorative, suppurative and tonic. Useful in abdominal pains, asthma, bronchitis, dysuria, oedema, epilepsy, gastric and duodenal ulcer, skin diseases and sore throat.	Anti-oxidant, anxiolytic. Side effects- oedema, hypertension and weight gain.
Gmelina arborea Roxb. (Verbenaceae)	Sriparni (S), Shivan (G).	Leaves and bark.	Demulcent, stomachic-tonic, refrigerant, alterative, laxative and galactagogue.	Ingredient of Dashmoolarisht.
Hedychium spicatum Ham. ex Sm. (Scitaminaceae)	Gandh-palasi (S), Kapur kachli (G, H, M).	Rhizom-es	Aromatic, anti-arthritic, appetizer, cardiac, stimulant, carminative, deodorant, denitrifice, emmenagogue, expectorant, febrifuge and tonic. Useful in colic, asthma, diarrhoea, dropsy, rheumatism, vomiting.	----
Helicteres isora Linn.(Sterculiaceae)	Avartani (S), Merdasingi (G), Murudseng (M), Marodfali (H), Screw Tree (E).	Root bark, fruits.	Stomach disorders, otorrhoea, ulcers in the ear, sore eyes and diabetes, amoebiasis.	----
Hemidesmus indicus (Linn.) R. Br. (Periplocaceae)	Sariva (S), Anantmul (G), Indian Sarsaparilla (E).	Root, flowers, leaves.	Alterative, antiabortive, antidiarrheal, anti-dysenteric, antipoisonous, aphrodisiac, appetizer, blood purifier, carminative, demulcent, diaphoretic, diuretic, expectorant, febrifuge, stomachic and tonic.	Antihistaminic.
Hibiscus rosa-sinensis Linn. (Malvaceae)	Japa (S), Jasud (G). Jabakusum (M), Shoeflower (E).	Flowers	Refrigent, emmollient, demulcent, aphrodisiac and emmenagogue, menorshagia, hair tonic.	----
Holarrhena antidysenterica Wallich.(Apocynaceae) *Holarrhena pubescens* Wallich. ex D. Don.	Kutaj (S), Indrajav (G), Kuda (M), Kareya (H)Kurchi Plant (E).	Bark and Seeds.	Anthelmintic, antidote to poison, antiperiodic, aphrodisiac, tonic, astringent, bitter, carminative, expectorant, febrifuge, antilithic. Cures amoebic dysentery, anaemia, asthma, bile and bowel complaints, broncho-pneumonia, colitis,	----

Linum usitatissimum Linn. (Linaceae)	Nil pushpi (S)Alsi (G), Linseed (E).	Seeds.	Demulcent, expectorant, diuretic, aphrodisiac, tissue relaxation.	Cardiac tonic, anticholesterol.
Luffa acutangula (Linn.) Roem. (Cucurbitaceae)	Mrudang-phala (S), Kadvitora (G)	Fruits, seeds.	Dropsy, splenitis, hemorrhoids and leprosy, eye troubles, delirium, diabetes.	——-
Luffa echinata Roxb. (Cucurbitaceae)	Dev-dali (S), Kukadvel (G), Devdali (M), Bamdal (H).	Whole plant.	Emetic and cathartic.	Splenomegaly, hepatomegaly wound healing.
Madhuca indica Muell.-Arg. (Sapotaceae)	Madhuca (S), Mahudo (G), Indian butter tree (E).	Stem bark, seeds, leaves, flowers.	Antiarthritic, antibilious, appetizer, astringent, cooling, detergent, emollient, nutritive, sedative, suppurative, tonic. Cures itches, bleeding gums, leprosy, skin diseases, diabetes, cold and cough.	——-
Mallotus philippensis (Koen.) MacBr. (Euphorbiaceae)	Rakta-fal (S), Kapilo (G), Kamala Dye (E).		Anthelmintic, anti-oxidant, aphrodisiac, astringent, bitter, blood purifier, cathartic, emollient, litholyptic, styptic and suppurative. Bile troubles, enlarged glands and boils, eruptions of skin, pimples and freckles.	——-
Mangifera indica Linn. (Anacardiaceae)	Amraphal (S), Ambo (G), Aam (M), Amb (H), Mango Tree (E).	Whole Plant.	Anthelmintic, anti-scorbutic, aphrodisiac, appetizer, astringent, cardiac, carminative, demulcent, diuretic and laxative. Cures debility of stomach, haemorrhage, heat strokes, leucorrhoea, menorrhagia, scabies and cutaneous affections.	——-
Maytenus emarginata (Willd.) Dinghou. (Celastraceae)	Vikamkat (S), Vikalo (G), Yekar (M), Baikal (H).	Leaves, fruits.	Antilithic, blood purifier, carminative, diuretic, febrifuge, laxative. Cures affections of bladder and uterus, burning sensations, calculous affections, colic, enlargement of abdominal viscera, increase secretion of bile, scrofulous affections, rheumatism and urinary disorders.	——-

Heine.(Acanthaceae)	[illegible]	Whole Plant.		
Hymenodictyon orixense (Roxb.) Wall. (Rubiaceae)	Bhamarchhallii (S), Bhamarchhal (G), Bhourchhal (M), Bhoulan (H).	Bark	Appetizer, digestive and intermittent fever.	——-
Hyocyamus niger Linn. (Solanaceae)	Parasikayamani (S), Khursani ajwain (H).	Dried leaves, flowers	Anodyne, anthelmintic, anti-aphrodisiac, antiseptic, astringent, cardiac, carminative, expectorant, hypnotic, narcotic, sedative and Stomachic. Useful in cephalic trouble, colic, insanity, insomnia and irregular menses.	——-
Indigofera tinctoria Linn. (Fabaceae)	Neelam (S), Gadi (G), Neel (M), Guli (H), Indigo Plant (E).	Roots, fruit color.	Useful in epilepsy, sores and bronchitis, antidote to arsenic poison, rheumatism, leprosy, hydrophobia, palpitation of heart and dropsy.	Anti-oxidant. Spleen and liver ailment.
Ipomoea digitata Linn. (Convolvulaceae)	Kshirvidari (S, G).	Roots.	Nutritional and useful in debility and sterility as well as good antacid.	——-
Ipomoea nil (L.) Roth. (Convolvulaceae)	Kalaunnika (S), Kaladana (G), Pharbities Seeds (E).	Dried seeds.	Attenuant, anthelmintic, blood purifier, diuretic, purgative, emmenagogue, fever, phlegm, bile and melancholy, rheumatism, hepatic stimulant.	——-

Melia azedarach Linn. (Meliaceae)	Maha-Nimb (S), Bakanlimbdo (G), Kadunimb (M), Bakain (H). Persian lilac (E).	Whole plant.	Useful in skin diseases rheumatoid arthritis, wounds and worms, leucoderma, syphilis, jaundice and fever.	----
Mentha piperita Linn. (Lamiaceae)	Putina (S), Fudino (G), Pudima (H), Pudherna (M), Wild Mint (E).	Leaves	Carminative and spasmolytic.	Heals Ulcers
Merremia turpethum (L.) Shah and Bhatt.(Convolvulaceae) *Operculina terpethum*	Trivvruta (S), Nasotar (G), Nisotar (M), Nisoth (H). Turpeth (E).	Roots, leaves.	Rheumatism, piles, swellings, urinary disorders and improves vitality.	Only black nasotar in purgative. Jalap substitutes nisoth. Black nasotar could be cultivated. JALAP- *Mirabilis jalapa*.
Mesua ferrea Linn. (Clusiaceae)	Nagkesar (S, G, H).	Flowers, buds, bark.	Anthelmintic, aphrodisiac, astringent, cardiac, carminative, diuretic, expectorant, stomachic and sudorific. Useful in asthma, cough, bleeding piles, dysentery, rheumatism, impotency and leucorrhoea, menorrhagia, epistatis.	----
Michelia champaca Linn. (Magnoliaceae)	Swarnachampak (S), Pilo-champo (G), Champa (H), Sonachafa (M).	Bark and flowers.	Indicated in rheumatoid arthritis, burning syndrome, as blood purifier, urticaria, anthelmentic, in spasmodic dismenorrhoea, malarial fever. Also useful in nausea, renal diseases, delirium.	----
Mimusops elengi Linn. (Sapotaceae)	Bakool (S), Borsallii (G), Mulsari (H), Barsali (M).	Bark, flowers, seeds.	Controls discharges from bladder and urethra, anguina, helps to promote childbirth, increase fertility, antidote, hydrophobia and insanity, pyorrhea, spongy gum.	----
Momordica charantia Linn. (Cucurbitaceae)	Karvellii (S), Karela (G, H). Bitter Gourd (E).	Leaves, fruits and root.	Malignant ulcers, skin affections, gout, rheumatism, liver and spleen diseases, melancholia, leprosy and piles.	Diabetes. Juice contr-aindicated in pregnancy.

Moringa oleifera Sm.(Moringaceae)	Shigru (S), Saragavo (G), Shegta (M), Sahimjna (H). Horse Radish Tree (E).	Root bark, flowers, seed oil.	Abortifacient, anthelmintic, antilithic, carminative, digestive, diuretic, emmenagogue, rubifacient, stomachic, stimulant. Useful in burns, bleeding piles, constipation, dysentery, scalds.	Splenomegaly, ringworm. Contraindicated- pregnancy. Leaf juice has broad-spectrum anti-bacterial activity.
Mucuna prurita Hook. f. (Fabaceae)	Kapikachu (S), Kavanch (G), Kuyeli (M), Kaunch (H). Cowhage Plant (E).	Seeds, root, fruit.	Anthelmintic, aphrodisiac, astringent, diuretic, nervine tonic. Useful in cholera, dropsy, leucorrhoea, tonic and seminal weakness.	Rheumatoid arthritis. Contains L-Dopa, useful in Parkinsonism.
Myrica esculenta Ham. ex Don. (Myricaceae)	Somvalk (S), Kaiphal, Katphal, Kaphal (G, H, M). Bay Berry (E).	Dried bark of the root.	Alterative, antiseptic, aromatic, astringent, carminative, dentifrice, diaphoretic, resolvent, stimulant and tonic. Indicated in asthma, catarrh, cough, diarrhoea, earache, fever, gonorrhoea, throat infections and piles.	——-
Nardostachys jatamansi (Don.) DC.(Valerianaceae)	Jatamansi (S, G, H), Balchir (M), Indian Spikenard (E).	Dried rhizome and roots.	Antiseptic, appetizer, aromatic, carminative, deobstruent, diuretic, emmenagogue, expectorant, nervine tonic, spinal sedative, stimulant, tonic, tranquilizer and vermifuge. Indicated in blood pressure, cough, diabetes insipidus, diarrhoea, respiratory disorders, dysmenorrhoea, epilepsy, erysipelas, flatulence, hysterical convulsions, leprosy, and palpitation of heart.	Hepato protective activity reported.
Nelumbo nucifera Gaertn. (Nelumbonaceae)	Pankaj, Ambuja (S), Kamal (G) Lotus (E), Kanval(H).	Whole plant	Urine retention and cough. Astringent, cardiac, conceptive, cooling, demulcent, diuretic, refrigent. Used in cholera, diarrhoea, vomiting, mennorrhagia, skin diseases, nervous exhaustions.	——-
Nerium indicum Mill.(Apocynaceae)	Karvir (S), Lal- Karen (G), Kanher (M), Kaner (H), Oleander (E).	Root and Root Bark	Anthelmintic, cardiac, carminative, diaphoretic, febrifuge. Useful in curing swellings, leprosy, skin diseases, ulcers and cancer.	Poisonous in large doses.

Nyctanthes arbortristis Linn.(Oleaceae)	Parijatak (S), Parijat (G), Night Jasmine (E) Khurasali(M)	Leaves	Sciatica, eye diseases, constipation, scurvy febrifuge.	----
Ocimum sanctuminn (Lamiaceae)	Vrunda (S), Tulsi (G, H), Tulasa (M), Holy Basil (E).	Leaves, seeds Roots.	Anticatarrh, demulcent, diaphoretic, digestive, diuretic, expectorant, febrifuge, stomachic. Useful in bronchitis, catarrhal fever, hepatic infection, skin diseases, aphrodisiac coolant.	Hypoglycemic, immuno-modulator, radio protective, anti-tumour property. Contraindicated in pregnancy.
Oroxylum indicum (L.) Venten. (Bignoniaceae)	Tintuk, Shyonak (S), Tetu (G, M), Sonapatha (H).	Root Bark.	Highly effective in diarrhoea and dysentery. Analgesic, anti-inflammatory. Good drug for rheumatoid arthritis.	One of the ingredients of dasamularisht.
Pandanus odoratissimus Lam.(Pandanaceae)	Ketki (S), Kevado (G), Kevada (H), Swetkevada (M), Screw Pine (E).	Roots, fruits, flowers.	Abortifacient, antiseptic, aphrodisiac, carminative, cephalic, deodorant, stomachic. Constipation, debility, headache, hysteria, skin diseases, strengthens the heart and liver.	Used in debility (New activity).
Papaver somniferum L. (Papaveraceae)	Ahifen (S), Afin (G), Afim (M, H), Poppy Seeds, Opium (E).	Seeds, exudute, fruits..	Analgesic, anaesthetic, anticolic, antidiuretic, astringent, depression of cerebrum, diaphoretic, expectorant, febrifuge, hypnotic, induction of nausea, narcotic and sedative.	Highly narcotic strong anti-diarrhoeral.
Pedalium murex Linn. (Pedaliaceae)	Bruhat-gokshru (S), Moto-gokhru (G), Badagokhru (H), Monthegokhru (M).	Whole plant, fruits	Impotence, genito-urinal disorders, leprosy, rheumatism, diuretic, Spermatorshoea, renal colic, oligospermia.	Dose- churna- 3 g.
Phyllanthus emblica Linn. (Euphorbiaceae)	Dhatari (S), Amla (G), Avla (M), Aonla (H), Indian Gooseberry (E).	Fruits.	Refrigent, diuretic, antiscorbutic and laxative. Cooling, digestive, anti-oxidant and astringent.	Ingredient of triphala and Chyavanprash. Tonic.
Phyllanthus fraternus Webst. (Euphorbíaceae)	Tamlaki (S), Bhoyamli (G), Bhuiavla (M, H). Katuka (S), Kadu (G),	Whole plant.	Anti-viral, deobstruent, sweet, cooling, blood purifier, cures itching.	Hepato-protective.

Picrorrhiza kurroa (Scrophulariaceae)	Kutki (H), Kutaki (M).	Rhizom-es, roots.	Cholagogue, immuno-stimulant, slow intermittent fever, asthma, ascitis.	Anti-oxidant. Contrain-dicated- hepatitis.
Pinus roxburghi Sarg. (Coniferae)	Saral (S), Chir (H).	Resin called as Pine resin.	Appetizer, anthelmintic, antispasmodic, cardiac, carminative, diaphoretic, diuretic, expectorant. Useful in diarrhoea, dysentery, fainting and ulcerations.	----
Piper longum Linn. (Piperaceae)	Pippali (S),Lindipipar (G), Pippali (H), Pimpli (M), Black Pepper (E).	Dried Fruits, leaves.	Alexipharmic, antiperiodic, digestive, diuretic, stimulant, fever, dysentery, cough, hysteria, cholera, dyspepsia, piles, aphrodisiac.	Anti-fibromyalgia syndrome (New activity).
Piper nigrum Linn. (Piperaceae)	Marich (S), Kalamari (G), Kalimirch (H, M), Black Pepper (E).	Dried fruits.	Anticonvulscent, bioenhancer, appetizer, used in viral hepatitis, anti-histaminic, counterirritant, anti-flatulent..	----
Pistacia integrifolia (Stew.) Rech. f. (Pistiaceae)	Shrungi (S), Kakadsingi (G) Kakrasingi (M, H)	Fruit.	Appetizer, expectorant and tonic. Useful in asthma, cough, chronic pulmonary affections, diarrhoea, dysentery and dyspepsia, loss of appetite, phthisis, psoriasis and vomiting.	----
Plantago Ovata Forsk(Plantaginaceae)	Aswagol (S), Ghodajceru, Ishabgol (G), Ishabgol, Blond Psyllium (E).	Dried seeds, husk.	Aphrodisiac, cooling, emollient, demulcent, diuretic, expectorant, chronic diarrhoea, constipation, rheumatism, gout, highly mucilaginous.	Very safe laxative as well as anti-diarrhoeal.
Pluchea lanceolata Clarke. (Asteraceae)	Shreyasi (S), Rasna (G, M, H).	Root, Leaves, Whole Plant.	Indicated in rheumatism and gastritis.	----
Plumbago zeylanica Linn. (Plumbaginaceae)	Chitrak-mula (S), Safed chitro (G), Chitrak (M), Chita (H), Leadwort (E).	Roots, leaves	Dyspepsia, piles, anasarca, diarrhoea, skin diseases, abortifacient, as a styptic in post partum haemorrhages, useful on leucoderma along with cow's milk.	At times blister forming.

Pongamia pinnata (L.) Pierre. (Fabaceae)	Karanja (S), Kanji (G), Karanj (M, H), Indian Beech (E).	Leaves, bark, seed oil.	Alterative, antiseptic, astringent, carminative, cooling, stimulant. Used in diabetes, diarrhoea, dyspepsia, epilepsy, insanity, and herpes.	Oil is highly effective on skin diseases and backache. Equitable with diesel.
Prosopis cineraria Linn. (Mimosaceae)	Agni-garbh (S), Khijado (G), Sami (M), Chikur (H). Spung tree (E).	Fruits. Leaves. Galls, Gum.	Demulcent and pectoral.	Asacred tree.
Psoralea corylifolia Linn. (Fabaceae) *Cullen corylifolia*	Bakuchi (S), Bavachi (G), Bapchi Seeds (E).	Seeds.	Laxative, stimulant, aphrodisiac, anthelmintic, leucoderma, skin diseases.	——-
Pterocarpus marsupium Roxb. var *acerifolium*.(Fabaceae)	Bijak (S), Biyo (G), Indian kino, malabar kino (E).	Leaves, flowers, bark gum	Phlegm, leprosy, sore eyes, gonorrhoea, haemorrhage, rheumatism and constipation. Improves vitality and complexion.	Anti-diabetic.
Pueraria tuberosa DC. (Fabaceae)	Vidarika (S), Bhoykolu (G), Bilai kand (H), Bhui kohla (M).	Tubers.	Aphrodisiac, cardiac, diuretic, emetic, expectorant, febrifuge, lactagogue, refrigerent and tonic. Used in swellings, constipation, debility, rheumatoid arthritis, sore throat and vomiting.	——-
Punica granatum Linn. (Punicaceae)	Dadima (S), Dadam (G), Dalimb (M), Anar (H), Pomegranate (E).	Root bark, leaves, flowers	Anthelmintic, astringent, cardiac, cooling, diuretic, expectorant, refrigerent, suppurative, diarrhoea, dysentery. Increases seminal flow.	——-
Rauwolfia serpentina (Linn.) Benth. ex Kurz. (Apocynaceae)	Sarpagandha (S, G, H), Adkai (M), Rauwolfia (E).	Dried roots.	Anthelmintic, antidote to snake venom, depressant, expectorant, tonic, febrifuge, hypnotic. Cures insanity, insomnia, and high blood pressure.	——-
Rheum australe G. Don.(Polygonaceae)	Amlaparni (S), Revand-chini (H), Rhubarb (E).	Roots, dried rhizomes	Aperient, astringent, diuretic, emmenagogue, expectorant, purgative, stomachic and tonic. Useful in cough, diarrhoea, dysentery, jaundice, urino-genital troubles.	Specific for infantile indigestion.

Ricinus communis Linn.(Euphorbiaceae)	Arend (S), Divel (G), Arendi (M), Arendum (H), Castor Oil Plant (E).	Leaves, Roots and Seed oil.	Highly purgative and effective in rheumatism.	Hepato-protective, contraceptive.
Rosa centifolia. (Rosaceae)	Taruni (S), Gulab (G), Rose Plant (E).		Cardiac, blood purifier, cooling, astringent, refrigent, hyperchlorhydria.	— — —
Rubia cordifolia Linn.(Rubiaceae)	Manjistha (S, G), Manjith (H), Manjistha (M), Madder root (E).	Roots	Alexipharmic, alterative, antidysenteric, anthelmintic, astringent, carminative, deobstruent, emmenagogue, expectorant, febrifuge and tonic. Useful in cough, freckles of skin, ulcers, mental agony and paralytic affections.	— — -
Saccharum officinarum Linn. (Poaceae)	Ikshu-kand (S), Serdi (G), Sugarcane (E).	Juice from the leaves. Stem, roots.	Aphrodisiac, diuretic, laxative, tonic, biliousness, blood dysentery, bleeding piles, burning sensation, haemorrhagic diathesis, indigestion, leucorrhoea, strangury, phthisis, vasical calculi.	— — -
Salvadora persica Linn. (Salvadoraceae)	Piludi (S, G, M), Chota Pilu (H), Tooth brush tree (E). Meshwak.	Leaves, fruit oil, roots.	Fevers and amenorrhoea, antidote to all poisons, rheumatism, asthma, cough, spongy gum.	Seed yield oil useful on paralysis and muscular debility.
Santalum album Linn.(Santalaceae)	Bhadrasri (S), Chandan (G), Sandal wood tree (E).	Heart wood.	Bitter, cooling, sedative, astringent, genito-urinary and bronchial diseases, diuretic, expectorant, stimulant.	Wood oil highly priced, useful in cosmetics and perfumes.
Sapindus laurifolius Vahl. (Sapindaceae)	Fanil (S), Aritha (G), Rithya (M), Ritha (H),Soap Nut Tree (E).	Root, leaves, fruits	Emetic, hernia, fits produced due to insensibility.	— — -
Saraca asoca (Roxb.) de Wilde. (Caesalpiniaceae)	Yamal-patrak (S), Ashok (G, M, H). Ashok Tree (E).	Dried bark.	Astringent, uterine sedative in menorrhagia. Cures dysmenorrhoea, fibroids.	— — -

Semecarpus anacardium L. f.(Anacardiaceae)	Agnimukh (S), Bhilamo (G), Biba (M), Bhilava (H), Marking Nut Tree (E).	Seed, Fruit.	Stimulant, narcotic, digestive, alterative, nervine tonic severe escharotic to be handled carefully. Contraindicated for bilious patients, anti-carcinazenic.	----
Sesamum indicum Linn. (Pedaliaceae)	Krishna-til (S), Til (G, M, H), Gingilly, Sesamum (E).	Leaves, flowers, seeds.	Aphrodisiac, anti-arthritic, demulcent, dysentery, emollient, emmenagogue, expectorant, lactagogue, styptic, tonic. Useful in burns, bleeding piles, constipation, cough, dysentery, scalds, urinary complaints, abortifacient.	Dental problems.
Sesbania grandiflora Pers. (Fabaceae)	Munipushpa (S), Agathio (G), Agastha (M), Hathiya (H).	Root, flowers, leaves, bark.	Cooling, febrifuge and astringent. Soothing spasmodic pain. Rich in Vitamin A, useful in night blindness.	Root paste mixed with datura root is highly effective in inflammation.
Sida cordifolia Linn.(Malvaceae)	Bala (S, G), Khareti (H), Khirhanti (M), Indian Mallow (E).	Whole plant	Demulcent, emollient. Useful in Gout, bleeding piles, rheumatism, pulmonary tuberclosis, swellings and as tonic. To treat post-partum infections	Root with cow milk useful in facial palsy. Adaptogenic and immunostimulant. Side effects- lathargia and pyloric obstructions.
Solanum nigrum Linn. (Solanaceae)	Kakmachi (S), Piludi (G), Black Nightshade (E).		Cough, skin diseases, rheumatism and gout, chronic enlargement of liver, eye diseases. Highly effective in vertigo and nausea.	Hepatoprotective.
Solanum xanthocarpum Burm. f. (Solanaceae)	Kantakari (S), Bhoyringni (G), Bhuiringni (M), Kanteri (H), Wild Egg Plant (E).	Dried Whole Plant. Dried roots	Alterative, anthelmintic, carminative, demulcent, diuretic, emmenagogue, expectorant, febrifuge. Used in anasarca, asthma, blood cancer, bronchitis, catarrhal fever, chest pain, cough, dysentery, dysuria, rheumatism and vomiting.	Anti-cancer.
Sphaeranthus indicus Linn. (Asteraceae)	Mundi-tika (S), Mundi (M, H), Gorakh-mundi (G).	Whole Plant.	Indicated in indigestion, worms, elephantiasis, cough, asthma and leucoderma.	----
Sterculia urens Roxb.(Sterculiaceae)	Kadayo (G).	Gum	Highly effective in throat affections.	----

Stereospermum suaveolens (Roxb.) DC. (Bignoniaceae)	Patala (S), Padad (G).	Leaves.	Useful in chronic dyspepsia, asthma, blood purifier, swellings, cough and vomiting.	One of the ingredients of dasamularisht.
Strychnos nux-vomica Linn.(Loganiaceae)	Vistinduk (S),Jherkachoru (G), Kuchla (H), Kajra (M). Nux-vomica (E).	Seeds.	Alexipharmic, aphrodisiac, appetizer, antiperiodic, cardiac stimulant, digestive, diuretic, emmenagogue, febrifuge, nervine tonic, purgative, stomachic. Indicated in anaemia, bronchial asthma, chlorosis, diabetes, debility, dysentery, pulmonary dyspnoea and intermittent fever.	One of the most important medicine in Homoeopathy. Dose- extract – 0.25 to 2.0 gms, tincture – 5 to 20 drops.
Swertia chirayita (Roxb. ex Flem.) Karsten. (Gentianaceae)	Kirat-tikta (S), Chiraita (H), Kirayat (M), Chirayata (E).	Whole plant.	Alterative, anthelmintic, bitter, carminative, digestive, expectorant, febrifuge, laxative, stomachic and tonic. Useful in asthma, bilious affections, constipation, diarrhoea, dyspepsia, flatulent, malarial fever and skin diseases.	Anti-inflammatory, immuno-stimulant, anti-oxidant activity reported.
Symplocos racemosa (Thunb.) Miq. (Symplocaceae)	Lodhra (S, G), Lodh (H).	Bark	Absorbent, alterative, antidropsical, anti-leprotic, astringent, blood purifier, dentifrice, expectorant, febrifuge, haemostatic, ophthalmic, refrigerant, resolvent, stomachic, styptic and suppurative.	——-
Syzygium aromaticum Linn. (Myrtaceae)	Devkusum (S), Lavang (G, M), Loang (H), Clove (E).	Dried flower buds.	Carminative, stomachache, anti-emetic.	Anti-herpes, anti-thrombic and anti-oxidant.
Syzygium cumini (L.) Merr. and Perry.(Myrtaceae)	Jambu (S, G,)Jamun (H), Black Berry (E).	Fruits Leaves Bark.	Astringent, carminative, diuretic, febrifuge and stomachic. Used in diarrhoea, dysentery, indigestion, leucorrhoea, against ringworms, anti-diabetic.	——-
Tamarindus indica Linn. (Caesalpiniaceae)	Amlika (S), Amli (G).Tamarind (E).		Anodyne, aperient, astringent, diuretic, febrifuge and tonic.	

Tamarix gallica. (Tamaricaceae)	Patra-vash (S), Padvash (G), Faras (M, H), Mayafal (E).	Galls	Indicated in cough, brachycardia, anaemia, useful in sexual debility.	----
Tecomella undulata (Sm.) Seem. (Bignoniaceae)	Rohitak (S), Ragat-rohido (G), Rohida (M), Rohira (H).	Bark	Anthelmintic, antidote to poison, astringent, blood purifier, carminative, stomachic. Useful in eye troubles, indigestion, jaundice, leucorrhoea, piles and worms, tumours.	----
Tephrosia purpurea (L.) Pers. (Fabaceae)	Pli-hari (S), Sarpankho (G), Oonhali (M), Sarfanka (H). Purple Tephrosia (E).	Whole plant.	Deobstruent, diuretic, cough, asthma, scrofulous glands, enlargement of liver, spleen and kidneys, rheumatism, asthma and abscesses.	----
Terminalia arjuna (Roxb. ex DC). Willd. and Arn. (Combretaceae)	Indradaru (S), Arjunsadad (G), Arjuna (E).	Bark	Astringent, cooling, cardiac stimulant, blood purifier and anti-rheumatic.	----
Terminalia bellirica (Gaertn.) Roxb.(Combretaceae).	Bibhitak (S), Baheda (G), Behada (M)Behera (H), Beleric Myrobalan (E).	Dried ripe Fruits.	Astringent, tonic, expectorant, laxative, anti-rheumatic.	Constituent of triphala. Cures insomnia.
Terminalia chebula Retz. (Combretaceae)	Haritaki (S), Harde (G), Harad (H), Chebulic Myrobalan (E).	Dried mature Fruits.	Astringent, dentifrice, purgative, stomachic, tonic. Cures asthma, ulceration, dysentery, diarrhoea, fever and flatulence, piles, vomiting and worms.	----
Thespesia populnea (L.) Sol. ex Correa. (Malvaceae)	Parish (S), Paraspiplo (G), Paraspipal (M), Gujdund (H). Tulip tree (E).	Root bark, juice of flowers, seed oil.	Used in bruises, sprains, insect bites especially centipedes, scabies, sores and inflamed joints.	----
Tinospora cordifolia Miers. (Menispermaceae)	Amruta (S), Galo (G)Gulvel (M), Giloy (H).	Leaves and mature stem	Alterative, anthelmintic, anti-arthritic, anti-periodic, antipyretic, aphrodisiac, bitter tonic, blood purifier, cardiac, carminative, digestive,	Tonic. Anti-ulcer, anti-diabetic and anti-oxidant .

			diuretic, expectorant, febrifuge, nutritive and stomachic. Useful in Jaundice and idiopathic fever, palpitation of heart, kidney complaints.	
Trachyspermum ammi (Linn.) Sprague. (Apiaceae)	Ajmodika (S), Ajmo (G), Owa (M), Ajwain (H), Bishop's Weed Seed (E).	Seed.	Stimulant, stomachic, carminative, antispasmodic and antiseptic.	----
Tribulus terrestris Linn. (Zygophyllaceae)	Gokshur (S), Nanu-gokhru (G), Kante-gokhru (M), Chota-gokhru (H).	Fruits, roots, whole plant.	Alterative, anthelmintic, anti-arthritic, aphrodisiac, cooling, demulcent, expectorant, tonic, calculous affections, kidney diseases and urinary discharges.	----
Trichosanthes cucumerina Linn.(Cucurbitaceae)	Patol (S), Kadva-patoda (G), Katupadval (M), Vanpatal (H)	Whole plant	Alterative, anodyne, anthelmintic, blood purifier, cooling, cardiac, carminative, digestive, expectorant, febrifuge, hair tonic, laxative, purgative, stomachic and suppurative. Anasarca, ascites, bilious fever, boils, debility, fever and jaundice, antacid.	Skin diseases.
Trigonella foenum-graecum Linn.(Fabaceae)	Pit-bija (S), Methi (G)Fenugreek (E).	Seeds.	Aperient, aphrodisiac, astringent, carminative, demulcent, diuretic, emollient, suppurative. Used in cough, diarrhoea, dysentery, dyspepsia, dropsy, enlargement of spleen and liver, inflammatory affections, leucorrhoea, swellings.	----
Typha angustata Bory and Chaub. (Typhaceae)	Aerka (S), Ghabajariu (G), Ramban (M), Patiha (H).	Fruits, aerial bark	Useful in renal obstacles, burning syndromes, flowers antiseptic, stops bleeding.	Effective in healing of wounds.
Uraria picta Desv.(Fabaceae)	Chitra-parni (S), Pithavan (G), Ran-ganja (H), Shankarjata (M).	Whole plant.	Increases lactation after pregnancy, oxytocic, tonic and bleeding piles.	Bone fracture. Ingradient of Dashmoolarisht.

Urginea indica Linn.(Liliaceae)	Mukh-dushak (S), Vandungri (G), Indian Squill (E).	Fleshy inner part of the bulb.	Anthelmintic, cardiac stimulant, digestive, diuretic, emmenagogue, expectorant. Cures asthma, calculous affections, bronchitis, paralysis, and rheumatism.	——-
Vernonia anthelmintica (Linn.) Willd. (Asteraceae)	Van-jiraka (S), Kadujire (M), Kalijiri (G).	Dried Seeds.	Powerful anthelmintic property. Useful in leucoderma and other skin diseases, cough and flatulency.	——-
Vernonia cinerea (Linn.) Less. (Asteraceae)	Sahdevi (S, H), Sahadevi (G, M).	Root, Leaves, Whole Plant.	Useful in febrile affections, spasm of the bladder, strangury and elephantiasis.	——-
Viola odorata Linn.(Violaceae)	Banpsa (S), Banafshah (G, M, H).	Flowers, whole plant.	Aperient, antipyretic, cooling, demulcent, diaphoretic, diuretic, emetic, emollient, expectorant, febrifuge and purgative. Useful in asthma, bleeding piles, throat cancer, constipation, headache and skin diseases.	——-
Vitex negundo Linn.(Verbenaceae)	Nirgundi (S), Nagod (G), Mevadi (H), Nigad (M), Five leaved chaste (E).	Leaves	Anodyne, anti arthritic, appetizer, astringent, cardiac, cephalic, demulcent, emmenagogue, expectorant, febrifuge, nervine tonic. Useful in asthma, bladder irritation, catarrhal diarrhoea, dyspepsia, intestinal haemorrhage, sciatica, general fatigue.	——-
Withania somnifera (L.) Dunal. (Solanaceae)	Vajigandha (S), Aswagandha (G), Winter Cherry (E).	Dried roots.	Tonic, alterative, galactagogue, aphrodisiac, nervine sedative.	——-
Woodfordia fruticosa (Linn.) Retz. (Lythraceae)	Dhataki (S), Dhavadi (G), Dhavas (M), Dhay (H).	Roots, leaves, flowers.	Stimulant, astringent. Useful in skin diseases.	For anti-natal care.
Zingiber officinale Rosc. (Scitaminaceae)	Adaraka (S), Adu (G), Ginger root (E).	Rhizom-es	Anorexia, rheumatoid arthritis, dyspepsia, nausea.	——-
Zizyphus mauritiana Lamk. (Rhamnaceae)	Rajvadar (S), Bor (G), Gonamp (M, H), Chinese Date (E).	Bark, fruitsleaves	Digestive and blood purifier, fever and delirium, cachexia.	——-

Chapter–9

GLOSSARY OF MEDICAL AND PHARMACOLOGICAL TERMS

Explanatory Terms/Pharmacological Terms/Medical Terms

1. **ABORTIFACIENT** – An agent that promotes abortion.
2. **ABSCESS** – Localized collection of pus produced by pyogenic organisms.
3. **ACUTE MANIA** – Phase of manic-depressive psychosis in which the prevailing psychomotor over - activity and often pathological excitement prevails.
4. **ALEXIPHARMIC** – Word – Alexi., i.e. word blindness, an inability to interpret the significance of the printed or written word, but without loss of visual power or loss of ability to read. Resisting effects of poison or infection, antidote or prophylactic.
5. **ALTERATIVE** – A drug that corrects disordered process of nutrition and restores the normal functioning of organ or system.
6. **AMENORRHOEA** – Abnormal suppression of menses.
7. **AMOEBIC DYSENTERY** – Dysentery caused due to *Entamoeba histolytica.*
8. **ANAEMIA** – A deficiency of blood or of red blood cells or of the red colouring matter of the blood.
9. **ANALGESIC** – A drug that relieves pain.
10. **ANASARCA** – Subcutaneous liquid accumulation causing swelling.
11. **ANGINA** – Sense of suffocation or constriction. Angina pectoris- severe but temporary attack of cardiac pain that may radiate to arms. Mainly results myocardial ischaemia.
12. **ANODYNE** – A drug that relieves localized pain.
13. **ANOREXIA** – Literally means, no oxygen in the tissues. Usually used to signify hypoxia.
14. **ANTHELMINTIC** – A drug that acts against intestinal worms.
15. **ANTI-ABORTIVE** – Drug that prevents abortion.
16. **ANTI-ARTHRITIC** – A drug that cures or relieves arthritic pains and swellings.
17. **ANTI-BILIOUS** – Drug that provides relief against biliousness, i.e. general condition of indigestion, constipation, headache etc.

18. **ANTI-CANCEROUS** – Drug that counteracts cancerous growth of cells/tissues or any body part.
19. **ANTI-CATARRH** – Drug that acts against catarrh, i.e. mild inflammation of mucus membranes, especially of air passages in nose and throat.
20. **ANTI-COLIC** – Drug that relieves pain due to contraction of muscles in walls of intestines, caused by gas or other reasons.
21. **ANTI-DIARRHOEAL** – Drug that act on diarrhoeal infections, i.e. common gastro intestinal diseases.
22. **ANTIDOTE** – A remedy that counteracts or neutralizes the action of a poison.
23. **ANTI-DROPSICAL** – Drugs that acts/prevents/against dropsy, i.e. a leakage of the watery part of the blood into any of the tissues or cavities of the body.
24. **ANTI-LEPROTIC** – Describes any agent that prevents or cures leprosy.
25. **ANTI-LITHIATIC** – Drug that cures renal stones/ kidney stones.
26. **ANTI-LITHIC** – A drug that counteracts the development of stone or calculus.
27. **ANTI-MALARIAL** – Against Malaria.
28. **ANTI-OXIDANT** – Drug, which delays the process of oxidation.
29. **ANTI-PARASITIC** – Describes an agent that prevents or destroys parasites.
30. **ANTI-PERIODIC** – An agent that prevents the periodic return of a disease.
31. **ANTI-PHLEGMATIC** – Medicine affecting bronchial conjestion.
32. **ANTI-PHLOGISTIC** – One that relieves pain and inflammation.
33. **ANTI-PYRETIC** – Describes any agent that allays or reduces fever.
34. **ANTI-RHEUMATIC** – Describes any agent that prevents or lessens rheumatism.
35. **ANTI-SCORBUTIC** – A drug that prevents or cures scurvy, or a agent that supplements Vit. C to the body.
36. **ANTISEPTIC** – Chemical substance that destroy or inhibit the growth of micro-organisms. They can be applied to living tissues.
37. **ANTI-SPASMODIC** – Drug that cures spasmodic disorders.
38. **APERIENT** – A mild form of purgative.
39. **APHRODISIAC** – A drug that promotes sexual desire, Libido.
40. **APPETIZER** – Drugs that stimulates appetite.
41. **AROMATIC** – A fragrant, spicy and mildly stimulant drug.
42. **ASCITES** – Abdominal dropsy, accumulating liquid in visceral cavity.
43. **ASTHMA** – A chronic disorders of bronchial tubes.

44. **ASTRINGENT** – A drug that arrests secretion or bleeding.

45. **ATTENUANT** – An agent that renders microbes less virulent or that renders microbes ineffective

46. **BEDSORES** – Ulceration on any part of the body of bed-ridden patient.

47. **BERI - BERI** – A deficiency disease caused due to lack of vitamins, especially B1.

48. **BILE TROUBLES** – Bile is a thick bitter fluid secreted by liver; it is basically irregularity of secretion, because of several reasons.

49. **BILIOUSNESS** – Word usually used to signify vomit-containing bile.

50. **BLOOD DYSENTERY** – Inflammation of the bowel with evacuation of blood and mucus, accompanied by tenesmus and colic.

51. **BOWEL COMPLAINTS** – Word used to mention any disorders of large intestine.

52. **BRACHYCARDIA** – Slow rate of heart contraction, resulting in a slow pulse rate.

53. **BRAIN SEDATIVE** – Agent inducing sleep or soothing effects.

54. **BRONCHIAL AFFECTIONS** – Bronchial congestion coupled with / due to infections.

55. **BRONCHITIS** – Inflammation of bronchi with excessive production of mucus, cough and breathlessness.

56. **BRONCHO-PNUEMONIA** – A term used to describe a form of pneumonia in which, small areas of lungs are consolidated and distributed widely around bronchi and not in a lobal pattern. A windpipe swelling.

57. **BRUISES** – A discoloration of the skin due to an extravasations of blood into the underlying tissues; there is no abrasion of the skin.

58. **CACHEXIA** – A term denoting a state of constitutional disorder, malnutrition and general ill health. Chief signs of this condition are bodily emaciation, sallow unhealthy skin and heavy lusterless eyes.

59. **CALCULOUS AFFECTION** – A hard and solid concretion formed in the body, especially in the gall bladder, salivary duct or urinary organs.

60. **CANCER** – Any malignant growth of the cells of any part of the body where cells divides rapidly i.e. abnormal division.

61. **CARDIAC STIMULANT** – Agent that stimulates cardiac functioning.

62. **CARMINATIVE** – A drug that relieves flatulence.

63. **CATARRHAL AFFECTIONS** – Infection with or without inflammation of a mucous membrane with associated flow of mucus.

64. **CATARRHAL FEVER** – Fever associated with catarrhal infections / affections.

65. **CATARRH** – Chronic inflammation of mucous membrane with constant flow of thick sticky mucus.

66. **CATHARTIC** – A drug that induces active movements of the bowels (Large intestine).

67. **CEPHALIC** – Pertaining to the head, near the head; especially cephalic vein.

68. **CEREBRAL CONGESTION** – Any disorders pertaining with cerebrum or mal-functioning of cerebrum.

69. **CERVICAL ADENITIS** – Excessive tissue growth on cervix (neck).

70. **CHOLAGOGUE** – A drug that promotes flow of bile.

71. **CHOLERA** – An acute epidemic disease, caused by Vibrio comma. Main symptoms are the evacuation of copious 'rice water' stools accompanied by agonizing cramp and severe body collapse.

72. **CHOLITIS (COLITIS)** – Infection with or without inflammation of colon, may be acute or chronic often associated with ulcerative lesions. Colon is the large bowel extending from the caecum to the rectum.

73. **CHRONIC FEBRILE AFFECTIONS** – Unusual sickness accompanied with fever.

74. **CHRONIC ULCERATION** – loss of surface tissue, mostly dermal or mucosal loss.

75. **COLIC** – Pain due to spasmodic contraction of the abdomen.

76. **COLLYRIUM** – A lotion put in eyes for washing of eyes.

77. **COMPLEXION** – texture, color of the skin.

78. **CONCEPTIVE** – Helpful in conception.

79. **CONSTIPATION** – An implied chronic condition of infrequent and often differential evacuation of faeces due to insufficient food or fluid intake.

80. **CONTRACEPTIVE** – An agent used to prevent conception.

81. **CONVULSIONS** – Involuntary contractions of muscles resulting from abnormal cerebral stimulation.

82. **CONVULSIVE FITS** – Fits associated with convulsions, i.e. violent irregular motion of limb or body.

83. **CULINARY PURPOSES** – Useful for cooking and food preparation.

84. **CUTANEOUS AFFECTIONS** – Skin ailments.

85. **DEBILITY** – A condition of weakness with lack of muscle tone.

86. **DELIRIUM** – An extreme mental disturbance marked by excitement, restlessness and rapid succession of confused and unconnected ideas.

87. **DEMULCENT** – An agent having a soothing effect on the skin and mucous membrane.

88. **DENTIFRICE** – Dental cleaning agent e.g. tooth powder, tooth paste, chewing stick.

89. **DEOBSTRUENT** – A drug that removes an obstruction to secretion or excretion by opening the natural passages or pores of the body.

90. **DEPRESSANT** – Agents that causes depression.

91. **DIABETES** – Increase in blood sugar level, caused by the impaired secretion of insulin in the body.

92. **DIAPHORETIC** – A drug that induces copious perspiration.

93. DIARRHOEA – Deviation from regular bowel rhythm featured by an increase in frequency and fluidity of the stools.

94. DIATHESIS – A hereditary predisposition to a disease/ailment.

95. DIGESTIVE – Useful in digestion.

96. DIPTHERIA – An infectious disease of the throat and the air passage which become inflamed and swollen and are coated with a fibrinous exudates.

97. DIURETIC – A drug that increases the secretion and discharge or urine.

98. DROPSY – A disease marked by an excessive collection of a watery fluid in the tissues or cavities of the body.

99. DYSENTERY – An infectious disease of which the chief symptoms are acute diarrhoea and discharge of blood and mucus.

100. DYSMENORRHOEA – Usually painful and difficult menstruation.

101. DYSPEPSIA – Indigestion.

102. DYSPEPTIC AFFECTIONS – Ailments associated with infections coupled with dyspepsia, i.e. indigestion.

103. DYSURIA – Painful and difficult urination.

104. ECZEMA – A skin disease accompanied by swelling, redness and exudation of lymph.

105. ELEPHANTIASIS – A disease caused by a tiny worm and attended with hypertrophy of the affected parts.

106. EMETIC – A drug that induces vomiting.

107. EMMENAGOGUE – A drug that promotes menstruation or regulates the menstrual period.

108. EMOLLIENT – A drug that allays irritation of the skin and alleviates swelling and pain.

109. ENLARGEMENT OF LIVER – Commonly called as Hepatomegaly.

110. ENLARGEMENT OF SPLEEN – Commonly called as Splenomegaly.

111. EPILEPSY – A chronic nervous disorder marked by attacks of unconsciousness or convulsions.

112. EPISTAXIS – Bleeding from the nose.

113. ERUPTIONS OF SKIN – Any superficial infection or inflammation or even both of skin, i.e. acne, blisters, pimples and vesicants.

114. ERYSIPELAS – An acute, specific infectious disease with *Streptococcal* inflammation of the skin and subcutaneous tissues, accompanied by fever and constitutional disturbances.

115. ESCHAROTIC – An agent capable of destroying tissues to produce scar.

116. EOSINOPHILIA – Increased eosinophils in the blood. Eosinophils are type of polymorphonuclear leucocytes containing eosin-staining granules. Eosin is the red staining agent used in histology and laboratory diagnostic procedures.

117. EXPECTORANT – A drug that promotes the removal of catarrhal matter and phlegm from the bronchial tubes; alleviates coughing.

118. FACIAL PALSY – Paralysis of muscles supplied by the facial nerve.

119. FATIGUE – Term used in physiological experiments on muscle to denote diminishing reaction to stimulus applied.

120. FEBRIFUGE – An agent used for reducing fever.

121. FEBRILE AFFECTIONS – Infections or inflammations accompanied by fever. Common between ages of 6 months and 5 years.

122. FISTULOUS SORES – Boils and wounds associated with fistula. Fistula is a pipe like sore with a narrow opening.

123. FLATULENCE – A disorder in which there is an excessive collection of gas in the stomach.

124. FOMENTATIONS – A hot, wet application to produce hyperemia. Medical and surgical fomentation (poultice).

125. FRECKLES – Coloured spots on the exposed parts of the skin.

126. GALACTAGOGUE – A drug that promotes secretion and flow of milk.

127. GASTRITIS – Inflammation of the stomach, especially the mucous membrane lining.

128. GENITO URINAL DISORDERS – Pertaining to the reproductive and urinary organs.

129. GERMICIDAL – Agent that kills germs.

130. GLANDULAR ENLARGEMENT – Abnormal increase in size of any gland of the body.

131. GLANDULAR SWELLINGS – Local inflammations in the glands.

132. GONORRHOEA – An infectious venereal disease marked by an inflammation and discharge from the genital organs.

133. GOUT – A form of metabolic disorder in which sodium biurate is deposited in the cartilages of the joints, the ears and elsewhere. The big toe is characteristically involved and becomes acutely painful and swollen.

134. HAEMOPTYSIS – Spitting of blood from the lungs or bronchial tubes.

135. HAEMORRHAGE – Internal bleeding, especially profuse, from any part of the body like vessel, artery, capillaries etc.

136. HAEMORRHOIDS – Varicosity of the veins around the anus, external and internal types. The external one outside the anal sphincter, covered with skin, internal one inside the anal sphincter covered with mucous membrane.

137. HAEMORRHAGIC – The escape of blood from a vessel, arterial, capillary, venous designate the type of vessel from which it escapes.

138.HAEMOSTATIC – Any agent that arrests bleeding.

139.HEMICRANIA – Migraine coupled with headache especially one side of the head.

140.HEPATIC TONIC – Drug that relieves disorders or diseases of liver and helps it function properly.

141.HERNIA – Rupture; protrusion through its covering of any organ of the body.

142.HERPES – A deep-seated vesicular viral eruption causing neuralgic pains.

143.HICCUP – An involuntary inspiratory spasm of the respiratory organs, ending in a sudden closure of the glottis with the production of a characteristic sound.

144.HYDROCELE – Swelling due to accumulation of serous fluid in the tunica vaginalis of the testis or in the spermatic cord.

145.HYDROPHOBIA – Syn. Rabies.—Fatal infection in man caused by a virus; infection follows the bite of a rabid animal; e.g. dog, cat, fox, vampire bat. It is of worldwide distribution.

146.HYPERCHLORHYDRIA – Excessive hydrochloric acid in the gastric juice.

147.HYPOPROTHROMBINAEMIA – Deficiency of prothrombin in the blood, which retards its clotting ability.

148.HYSTERIA – A disease in which a physically healthy patient has lost control over acts and feelings and suffers from imaginary ailments.

149.HYSTERICAL CONVULSIONS – Neurosis usually arising from mental conflict and repression and characterized by the production of a diversity of physical symptoms. e.g. Fits, paralysis, anesthesia etc.

150.IMPOTENCY – Inability to participate in sexual intercourse, by custom referring to the male. It can be due to lack of sufficients number of sperms erection or premature ejaculation.

151.INFECTIONS – The successful invasion, establishment and growth of microorganisms in the tissues of the host. It may be of acute or chronic nature.

152.INFLAMMATION – The reaction of living tissues to injury, infection or irritation, characterized by pain, swelling, redness and heat. The degree of redness can be measured by tintometer.

153.INSANITY – Mental dearrangement, idiopathic psychic behaviour.

154.INSOMNIA – Stage of sleeplessness.

155.INTERMITTENT FEVER – Fever, which is marked by intervals of normal temperature between periods of rise of temperature.

156.INTESTINAL HAEMORRHAGE – Haemorrhage in intestines, i. e. bowels.

157.INTESTINAL WORMS – Infections caused by different types of worms in intestine.

158.INTOXICATING – State of being drunk; high excitement of elation. Drug that intoxicates.

159.ITCH – An infectious skin disease, caused by a mite, without specific lesions and marked by excessive itching; scabies.

160.JAUNDICE – A diseased condition in which there is a yellowish staining of the tissues and excretions with bile.

161.KIDNEY ACTIVATOR – Drug that activates or helps in proper functioning of kidney.

162.LACTAGOGUE – Galactagogue.

163.LAXATIVE – Drugs that produce peristalsis and promotes evacuations of the bowel, usually to relieve constipation.

164.LENITIVE – Capable of earing pain.

165.LEPROSY – A chronic wasting disease caused by a germ, the disease generally results in mutilations and deformities.

166.LEUCODERMA – A condition of the skin in which there is loss of melanin pigment wholly or partially resulting in white patches on the skin.

167.LEUCORRHOEA – A sticky, whitish vaginal discharge.

168.LITHOTOMY – Surgical removal of stones from the body.

169.LITHONTRIPTIC – A drug used for removing calculi or stones formed in the urinary system.

170.LUMBAGO – Rheumatism of the muscles especially back side of the body.

171.MALARIA – A recurrent disease marked by bouts of shivering, sudden rise of temperature and general aching of the body.

172.MALIGNANT ULCERS – Kind of ulcers that are virulent and dangerous and are likely to have fatal termination.

173.MELANCHOLIA (GROSS HUMOUR)– MELANCHOLIC A disorder of the mind marked by depression of spirits, self repentence and mental sluggishness.

174.MELANCHOLY – Term reserved in psychiatry to mean severe forms of depression.

175.MENORRHAGIA – Abnormally excessive menstruation.

176.MENSTRUAL SUPPRESSIONS – Any menstrual complaints; i.e., delay in the monthly discharge from uterus.

177.MYDRITIC – Drugs that cures mydriasis, i.e. abnormal dilation of the pupil of the eye.

178.NARCOTIC – A drug that induces deep sleep.

179.NAUSEA – A feeling of vomiting sensation.

180.NERVINE SEDATIVE – Drug that soothes or allays irritability of nervous systems.

181.NERVINE TONIC – Drug that rejuvenates nervous systems for proper functioning.

182.NERVOUS DEBILITY, NERVOUS DISORDERS, NERVOUS EXHAUSTIONS – Terms related to any disorders pertaining to nervous system. The disorders can be neuralgia, nervine sedations, etc and the drugs used are nervine stimulants, CNS depressants etc.

183.NEURALGIA – Pain felt along a nerve.

184.NEURALGIC – Drug that cures pain in the disturbed nerve

185.NOCTURNAL EMISSIONS – Involuntary discharge of the seminal fluid during the night.

186.NUTRITIVE – That provides nutrition.

187.OEDEMA – Abnormal infiltration of tissues with fluid. There are many causes- it can be in the blood or disease of the cardiopulmonary system, the urinary system and the liver.

188.OLIGOSPERMIA – Reduction in number of spermatozoa in the semen.

189.OPHTHALMIC – Pertaining to eye.

190.OPHTHALMIA – Inflammation of the eye, a type of conjunctivitis.

191.OTORRHOEA – A purulent discharge from the ear.

192.OXYTOCIC – Hastening parturition; an agent promoting uterine contractions.

193.OXYTOCIN – A hormone of pituitary gland causing contraction of the womb.

194.PALPITATION OF HEART – Beating of the heart of which the patient is conscious.

195.PARALYSIS – A disease in which there is loss of power of voluntary movement in any part of the body.

196.PHARYNGITIS – Inflammation of the pharynx.

197.PHLEGM – The secretion of mucus expectorated from the bronchi.

198.PILES – An inflamed condition of the veins in the anal region.

199.PNEUMONIA – Inflammation of the lungs.

200.PROPHYLACTIC – An agent that prevents disease.

201.PRURIGO – A chronic skin disease marked by the eruption of small, rounded, reddish pimples.

202.PSORIASIS – A common chronic inflammation of the skin, marked by rounded reddened patches, which are covered with dry silvery scales.

203.PHTHISIS – Term related to pulmonary tuberculosis.

204.PULMONARY AFFECTIONS – Infection with or without inflammations in the lungs or respiratory tube or both.

205.PULMONARY DYSPNOEA – A kind of lung and chest disorder.

206.PULMONARY TUBERCULOSIS – Infection & swelling of lungs due to bacterium, Mycobacterium tuberculosis (Koch's bacillus)

207.PURGATIVE – Drug causing evacuation of fluid faeces.

208.RECTAL FISSURES – Bruises on anal portion.

209.REFRIGENT – Drugs having cooling properties on surface of the body.

210.REFRIGERANT – A drug that relieves feverishness or produces a feeling of coolness.

211.RENAL STONES – Referred to as renal calculus, i.e. stone in the kidney.

212.RESOLVENT – Bringing amelioration.

213.RHEUMATISM – An indefinite term used for pains and swellings in the muscles, joints and certain tissues.

214.RHEUMATOID ARTHRITIS – A disease of unknown aetiology; characterized by a chronic polyarthritis mainly affecting the smaller peripheral joints, accompanied by general ill health and resulting eventually in varying degrees of crippling joint deformities and associated muscle wasting.

215.RINGWORMS – A parasitic skin disease usually marked by red, scaly, circular patches.

216.RUBEFACIENT – A mild counter-irritant.

217.SCABIES – An itching skin disease caused by a mite.

218.SCALDS – An injury caused by moist heat.

219.SCIATICA – An inflammation of the sciatic nerve at the back of the thigh.

220.SCROFULA – A disease of the lymphatic gland, often of the neck.

221.SCROFULOUS AFFECTIONS – Tuberculosis of bone or lymph gland.

222.SEDATIVE – A drug that reduces excitement, irritation and pain.

223.SEMINAL DEBILITY, SEMINAL WEAKNESS – Disorders pertaining to semen.

224.SINUSITIS – Inflammation of a sinus. Used exclusively for the paranasal sinuses.

225.SKIN ERUPTIONS – Kind of skin inflammation.

226.SORE EYES – Irritation in eyes due to boils and wounds in eyes. Sort of ophthalmic disorders.

227.SORE THROAT – Infection of throat in form of boils, irritation in throat.

228.SPASMS – Convulsive, involuntary muscular contraction.

229.SPERMATORRHOEA – Involuntary discharge of semen without orgasm.

230.SPLENITIS – Inflammation of the spleen.

231.STIMULANT – Syn. Stimulating, i.e. an agent that excites or increases function.

232.STOMACHACHE – Pain or unspecified disorders in stomach region. It can be cholera, diarrhoea or dysentery.

233.STOMELANCHOLICMACHIC – Agents, which increases appetite.

234.STRANGURY – Painful and drop-by-drop discharge of urine.

235.STYPTIC – An agent that checks bleeding.

236.SUDORIFIC – An agent, which induces sweating.

237. SUPPURATIVE – Agent that enhances the formation of pus.

238. SWELLINGS – Term used to describe local inflammations.

239. SYNOVITIS – Inflammation of synovial membrane.

240. SYPHILIS – A chronic venereal disease.

241. SYPHILITIC ULCERS – Ulcers in local lymph glands caused by Treponema pallidum.

242. THROAT AFFECTIONS – Inflammations with or without infection, or vice versa related to throat. It can be sore throat, gargle, catarrh, tonsillitis and diptheria.

243. TISSUE RELAXANT – Agents that relaxes tissues, i.e. reduces fatigue from tissues.

244. TONIC – Used to describe a state of continuous muscular contraction, as opposed to intermittent contraction. More specific is a drug that invigorates or improves the normal tone of an organ or the patient generally.

245. TONSILITIS – Inflammation of the tonsils.

246. TUBERCULOSIS – A specific infective disease caused by Mycobacterium tuberculosis. Many types such as pulmonary, miliary, avian, bovine etc., may occur.

247. TUMOUR – A mass of abnormal tissue which resembles the normal tissues in structure, but which fulfills no useful function and which grows at the expense of the body.

248. TYPHOID – An acute infectious disease characterized by ulceration of the intestines, eruption of rose-coloured spots and a typical course of temperature.

249. ULCERATION – Destruction of either mucous membrane or skin from whatever cause, producing a crater or indentation. It can be in blood vessel or in the lining of hollow organ.

250. ULCERS – An open sore on the body, mostly internal like peptic ulcers, gastric ulcers and duodenal ulcers.

251. URINARY SEDATIVE – Drug that soothes or allays irritability pertaining to any urinary tract disorders or infections.

252. URINO-GENITAL DISORDERS – Pertaining to the urinary and the genital organs.

253. URTICARIA – An allergic disease of systemic origin marked by painful and itching elevations of the skin.

254. VAGINAL INFECTIONS – Pertaining to vagina. Either vaginismus or vaginitis or both.

255. VERMIFUGE – A drug that expels intestinal worms.

256. VITILEGO – Skin disease of probable autoimmune origin characterized by areas of complete loss of pigment.

257. VISCERAL OBSTRUCTION – Obstruction of alimentary canal.

258. VOMITING – Ejection of the stomach contents through the mouth; sickness.

259. WHOOPING COUGH – An acute infectious disease featured by peculiar spasmodic attacks of coughing.

Chapter–10

GLOSSARY OF AYURVEDIC TERMS

1. **ADHIBHAUTIKA** – diseases caused by external physical factors like germs and accidents.
2. **ADHIDAIVEKA** – diseases caused due to seasonal, planetary and providential influences.
3. **ADHMANA** – Flatulence.
4. **ADHYATMIKA** – Spiritual state of mind that affects the body.
5. **ADISTHANA** – site of manifestation of a disease.
6. **AGANTUKA** – strange, exotic, outside influence.
7. **AGNI** – fire, one of the five elements that make up the universe; also refers to the enzymes of the body; digestive capability.
8. **AGNIVESHA** – sage Atreya's disciple who formulated the *Agnivesha Samhita.*
9. **AGNIVESHA SAMHITA** – ancient ayurvedic text said to be written in 1000 B. C.
10. **AHITA** – unhappy, miserable, sad
11. **AKASHA** – Sky one of the five elements.
12. **AMA** – a substance that accumulates in the joints due to improper digestion and causes rheumatism.
13. **AMAVATA** – rheumatism.
14. **ANANDAMAYA** – one of the five spiritual elements/layers that make up the individual, this helps in experiencing bliss.
15. **ANANTAVATA** – migraine.
16. **ANNAMAYA** – the physical body, one of the five layers of the individual.
17. **ANUMANA** – inference, deduction.
18. **ARISTHA** – medicated wine, a fermented decoction.
19. **ARKA** – distillate with the process of distillation
20. **ARTAVAJANANA** – that which promotes ovulation/menstrual flow.
21. **ARTHA** – wealth.

22. **ASAVA** – medicated wine.
23. **ASHTASHANA PARIKSHA** – eight fold method of medical examination used by ayurvedic physicians.
24. **ASTHI** – bone tissue.
25. **ASTIKA DARSHANA** – branch of Indian philosophy that recognizes the authority of the Vedas.
26. **ATHARVAVEDA** – one of the four vedic texts.
27. **ATISARA** – diarrhoea.
28. **ATMAN** – the soul, considered indestructible in Hindu philosophy.
29. **ATREYA** – ancient Hindu sage, one of the founding fathers of ayurveda.
30. **AVALEHA** – medicine in a thick viscous form, sort of marmalade.
31. **AYUR** – life.
32. **BALYA** – Imparting physical strength, increasing resistance to disease, immunity.
33. **BASTI** – Anema.
34. **BASTI ROGA** – disease of colour.
35. **BASTI SHODHANA** – said to cleanse the colour.
36. **BHARADVAJA** – ancient Hindu sage, one of the founders of ayurveda.
37. **BHEDANA** – purgation.
38. **BHEDANIYA** – purgative.
39. **BRAHMA** – the creator, one of the gods of the Hindu holy trinity. The other two are Shiva, the destructor and Vishnu, the preserver.
40. **BRAHMANS** – amongst Hindus, the class that by convention is supposed to comprise the educated priest; the knowledgeable.
41. **BRIMHANA** – nourishing therapy usually prescribed for old, emaciated and weak people. One of the six basic ayurvedic therapies.
42. **BUDDHI SMRUTI PRADA** – beneficial to intellect and memory.
43. **CHAKSHUSHYA** – beneficial to eyes.
44. **CHAPATI** – small round breads of coarse, unleavened dough eaten as an accompaniment in most Indian meals.
45. **CHARAKA** – ancient Hindu sage who wrote the most authoritative treaty on ayurveda *Charaka Samhita* based on *Agnivesha's teachings*.
46. **CHOORNA** – powder.
47. **DAHA** – burning sensation.

48. DAKSHA PRAJAPATI – according to Hindu legend, Brahma's son.

49. DANTA SHOOLA – toothache.

50. DARSHANA – a term of Indian philosophy; means visual observation in ayurvedic diagnosis; theoretical conceptualization.

51. DEEPAN – promoting digestive functions.

52. DHANVANTARI – the Hindu god of ayurvedic medicines.

53. DHARA – therapy involving the use of medicated oils.

54. DHARMA – in Hindu philosophy an individual' s role and duties in life, decided by his birth, class and occupation.

55. DHATUS – tissue elements of a living body, 7 dhatus are Ras, Rakta, Mansa, Meda, Asthi, Mujja and Shukra.

56. DINACHARYA – regimen prescribed by ayurveda to be followed during the day to prevent diseases and lead healthy life.

57. DOSHAS – basic functional units of the body. –three humours, according to ayurveda. They are Vat (Melancholic), Pitta (bilious) and Kafa (Phlegmatic).

58. DURGANDHYANASHANA – deodarant.

59. GARBHADA – promoting fertility/conception (in females).

60. GARBHASHAYYA SANKOCHAKA – oxytocic.

61. GARBHASHAYYOTTEJAKA – uterotropic.

62. GHEE – a clarified butter used widely in India both as a cooking medium and as a vehicle for many medicines.

63. GRIDHRASI – sciatica.

64. GRIVA SANDHIGATA VATA – cervical spondylosis.

65. GUNAS – basic attributes that characterize physical and psychological reality. There are three in all – *sattva, rajas, tamas.*

66. HIKKAANIGRAHAKA – that which controls hiccough.

67. HIKKAROGA – an attack of hiccups.

68. HITA – happy, good, beneficial.

69. HOMA – the act of offering oblations like pouring clarified butter into a sacred fire, an important ritual in Hindu worship.

70. HRIDROGA – heart disease.

71. JALA – water, one of the five elements.

72. JWARA – fever.

73. **KALPA** – literally, art. In this case, a galenical, a special formula.
74. **KAMA** – desire for love and sex.
75. **KAMALA** – jaundice.
76. **KAPHA** – phlegm, if roughly translated. According to ayurveda, one of the three doshas or basic units of the body. One of the 3 major types of personalities –phlegmatic.
77. **KAPHAJA** – that which originates from the imbalancing of kapha.
78. **KASA ROGA** – bronchitis, coughing.
79. **KASHYAPA** – one of the founding sages of ayurveda.
80. **KESHYA** – promoting healthy hair.
81. **KOSHAS** – successive layers of tissues that make up the individual.
82. **KRIMIJA** – disease caused due to external organisms, which enter the body. e.g intestinal worms.
83. **KSHAYA** – astringent taste and also decoction.
84. **KUSTHA** – dermatoses.
85. **LAGHU** – light, easy to digest.
86. **LANGHANA** – fasting that helps remove unwanted and poisonous matter from the body. One of the five basic ayurvedic therapies collectively called as Panchkarma.
87. **LAVAN** – salt and salty taste.
88. **LEKHANA** – weight reducing.
89. **LEPA** – medicinal paste for topical use.
90. **MADAKARAKA** – soporific.
91. **MADHUMEHA** – diabetes.
92. **MADHURA** – sweet taste.
93. **MAHABHUTA** – the basic elements that make up the universe. There are five in all- earth, water, fire, space (sky) and air.
94. **MAJJA** – bone marrow.
95. **MALAS** – human waste products that include stool, urine, perspiration, earwax, saliva.
96. **MAMSA** – muscle tissue.
97. **MANOMAYA** – one of the five layers that make up the individual; the psyche or what the individual thinks.
98. **MARGA** – route, way.
99. **MEDA** – fat.

100.MEDOROGA – obesity.

101.MOKSHA – ultimate salvation in Hindu philosophy that signifies freedom from the ceaseless cycle of birth and death.

102.MRIDU – soft, delicate, mild, gentle.

103.MUTRA – urine.

104.MUTRA JANANA – that which increases formation of urine.

105.MUTRA SAMGRAHANIYA – that which reduces urine output (antidiuretic).

106.MUTRALA – diuretic.

107.NADI PARIKSHA – pulse examination.

108.NASTIKA DARSHANA – branch of Indian philosophy that does not acknowledge the authority of the God.

109.NETRAHITA – beneficial to eyes.

110.NIDANA – diagnosis and prognosis put together.

111.NIDRAKA – sedative, hypnotic.

112.NIDRA – sleep.

113.OJAS – a substance formed during the metabolic transformation of tissue elements that is vital to the individual's survival as it provides immunity and supposed ora to the personality.

114.PAITTIKA – that which originates from pitta of bilious personality.

115.PANCHA MAHABBUTA – the five elements; prithvi, jal, agni, akash and vayu.

116.PANDU – anaemia.

117.PARASHARA – one of the ancient founding sages of ayurveda.

118.PARIKSHA – examination.

119.PARSHWASHULA – lateral chest pain.

120.PICHCHILA – sticky or viscous.

121.PITTA – one of the doshas- body humours. If loosely translated, it is bile.

122.PRADARAHARA – useful in menstrual and vaginal disorders.

123.PRAJASTHAPANA – that which promotes conception.

124.PRAKRITI – physical and psychological constitution of an individual. There are 3 basic personalities Vat (Melancholic), Pitta (bilious) and Kapha (Phlegmatic); there could be mixed combination too.

125.PRANAMAYA – one of the five layers that make up the individual. It is the layer, which enables an individual to feel and experience.

126.PRASHAN – to consume.

127.PRASHNA – to question or interrogate.

128.PRATYAKSHA – in person; form of ayurvedic examination in which the physician directly relies on his five senses; seeing, hearing, smelling, touching and tasting to diagnose a patient.

129.PRAVAHIKA – amoebic dysentery—resulting into watery stools.

130.PRAVAHIKAHARA – useful in dysentery.

131.PRITHVI – earth, one of the five elements of life.

132.PURVARUPA – the premonitory symptoms of a disease.

133.RAJAS – one of the three attributes of physical and psychological reality, rajas symbolizes energy and passion, other two are Tamas and Satva.

134.RAKTA – the red fraction of the blood.

135.RAKTA PITTA – bleeding diathesis.

136.RAKTA RODHAKA – haemostatic.

137.RAKTA SAMGRAHAKA – haemostatic.

138.RAKTA SHODHAKA – that which purifies blood.

139.RAKTA STAMBHAKA – that which controls bleeding.

140.RAKTA VARDHANA – that which increases blood.

141.RAKTA VIKARA – diseases of blood.

142.RASA – the plasma of blood excepting corpuscles; also lymph. The first material formation of the body after the food being assimilated.

143.RASAYANA – a therapy or a material that cause rejuvenation and reduces the effects of ageing.

144.RASONA KALPA – an intense and complex kind of rejuvenation therapy involving the use of garlic.

145.RATRICHARYA – regimen prescribed by ayurveda to be followed through the night to prevent diseases.

146.RECHANA – purgation.

147.RIGVEDA – one of the four vedic texts.

148.ROCHANA – stimulating appetite.

149.RUCHYA – that which stimulates taste.

150.RUKSHA – rough.

151.RUPA – the actual symptoms of a disease; external appearance of a patients.

152.SAMAVEDA – one of the four vedic texts, also a state of perfect health when all the three doshas are equally balanced in the body.

153.SAMPRAPTI – the way a disease is finally manifested in the body, symptomatology that helps in diagnosing ailment.

154.SANCHARA MARGA – the path through which disease spreads.

155.SANDHANIYA – uniting.

156.SANGYA STHAPANA – restoring consciousness.

157.SANNIPATA – the state in which all three doshas are imbalanced and the body is in imperfect health, also epileptic delirium.

158.SARA – fluid, liquid, cathartic.

159.SARAKA – possessing sara property.

160.SATTVA – one of the three attributes of reality, sattva signifies consciousness.

161.SHABDA – already existing statements about a disease made by experts based on their research, literally word, syllable that constitute knowledge.

162.SHEETA – cold.

163.SHONITASTHAPANA – that which promotes clotting.

164.SHOTHA – oedema.

165.SHUKRALA – promoting semen.

166.SHUKRAVRIDHIKARA – that which increases semen.

167.SHULA – colic, pain.

168.SHWITRA – vitilago.

169.SIDDHA DUGDHA – milk boiled with medicines.

170.SNEHANA – oleation therapy, also one of the six basic therapies. In this oil, ghee and even bone marrow is used.

171.SOOKSHMA – minute, subtle.

172.SPARSHANA – touch.

173.SROTA – channels of circulation that carry external nutrient matter to the body organs and remove metabolic waste, resources.

174.STAMBHANA – this is an astringent therapy that checks excessive physiological secretions, mostly retention during sexual intercourse.

175.STHANA – place.

176.SUSHRUTA – one of the founding sages of surgical procedures in ayurveda, he wrote the famous ayurvedic text *Sushruta Samhita.*

177.SWEDANA – one of the six basic therapies of ayurveda, this involves fomentation to induce perspiration.

178.TAILA – oil.

179.TAMAKA SWASA – bronchial asthma resulting into noisy, speedy, whizzing breathing.

180.TAMAS – one of the three basic attributes of reality, tamas signifies mass and stability.

181.UDARDA – urticaria.

182.UDBHAVA STHANA – site of origination of a disease.

183.UNANI TIBB – Greek-arabic medicine. This originated in ancient Greece and percolated to Arabian world between 8th to 13th centuries.

184.UNMADA – hysteria.

185.UPASAYA – an initial method to explore the nature of a disease, keeping in mind the symptoms and looking for possible diagnosis.

186.USHNA – hot, heating.

187.VATA – one of the three doshas or basic functional units of the body. Loosely translated as wind, melancholic, painful.

188.VATA SLAISHMIKA JWARA – influenza.

189.VATIKA – that which originates from vayu or vata.

190.VAYU – same as vata.

191.VEDA – ancient Aryan texts that contain the knowldege of Indian philosophy, religious practices, customs, modes of living etc. There are four vedic texts- Rig, Yajur, Sama and Atharva. These texts were compiled in a written form by disciples of Hindu sages from centuries of knowledge passed down orally. They are not the works of a single person.

192.VICHARCHIKA – eczema.

193.VIJNANMAYA – one of the layers that make up the individual, it signifies the intellect, which can discriminate between base and pure, right and wrong.

194.VRANA – ulcer, wound.

195.VRANAROPANA – that which promotes healing of wounds and ulcers.

196.VRANASHOTHA – inflammation.

197.VRANAVISHA – toxins from the wound.

198.VRISHYA – that which promotes virility.

199.VYATHA – pain, discomfort.

200.YAJURVEDA – one of the four vedic texts.

201.YAKRIT – liver.

202.YAKRITOTTEJAKA – liver stimulant.

203.YOGA – a form of physical exercises requiring extreme mental concentration, which according to Indian philosophy elevates the mind to a spiritual plane, thereby satisfying the demands of the body-mind-spirit complex.

204.YONIDOSHA – diseases of female reproductive system.

Chapter–11

LIST OF PLANTS AS PER B & H'S SYSTEM OF CLASSIFICATION

RANUNCULACEAE
Aconitum ferox (Bruhl.) Muk., *Aconitum heterophyllum* Wall. *Coptis teeta* Wall.
MAGNOLIACEAE
Michelia champaca Linn.
MENISPERMACEAE
Cissampelos pareira Linn. *Cocculus hirsutus* (Linn.) Diels. *Tinospora cordifolia* Miers.
PAPAVERACEAE
Argemone mexicana Linn. *Papaver somniferum* L.
(BRASSICACEAE) CRUCIFERAE
Lepidium sativum Linn.
CAPPARACEAE (CAPPARIDACEAE)
Crateava magna (Lour.) DC.
VIOLACEAE
Viola odorata Linn.
TAMARICACEAE
Tamarix gallica. , T Chinensis

MALVACEAE
Abelmoschus moschatus (L.) Medik. *Abutilon indicum* Sweet. *Hibiscus rosa-sinensis* Linn. *Sida cordifolia* Linn. *Thespesia populnea* (L.) Sol. ex Correa.
BOMBACACEAE
Bombax ceiba Linn.
STERCULIACEAE
Helicteres isora Linn. *Sterculia urens* Roxb.
LINACEAE
Linum usitatissimum Linn.
ZYGOPHYLLACEAE
Tribulus terrestris Linn.
RUTACEAE
Aegle marmelos Linn. *Limonia acidissima* Linn.
BALANITACEAE
Balanites aegyptaica (Linn.) Delile.
BURSERACEAE
Boswellia serrata Roxb. ex Colebr. *Commiphora wightii* (Arnott.) Bhandari.
MELIACEAE
Melia azaderach Linn.
Azadirachta indica Juss.
CELASTRACEAE
Celastrus paniculata Willd. *Maytenus emarginata* (Willd.) Dinghou.
RHAMNACEAE

Zizyphus mauritiana Lamk.
VITACEAE
Cissus quadrangularis Linn.
SAPINDACEAE
Cardiospermum helicacabum Linn. *Sapindus laurifolius* Vahl.
ANACARDIACEAE
Buchanania lanzan Spreng. *Mangifera indica* Linn. *Semecarpus anacardium* L. f.
MORINGACEAE
Moringa oleifera Sm.
FABACEAE (PAPILIONACEAE)
Abrus precatorius Linn. *Alhagi psuedalhagi* (M. Bieb.) Deav. *Butea monosperma* (Lamk.) Taub. *Clitorea ternatea* Linn. *Desmodium gangeticum* (Linn.) DC. *Dolichos biflorus* Linn. *Glycyrrhiza glabra* Linn. *Indigofera tinctoria* Linn. *Mucuna prurita* Hook. f. *Pongamia pinnata* (L.) Pierre. *Psoralea corylifolia* Linn. *Pterocarpus marsupium* Roxb. *Pueraria tuberosa* DC. *Sesbania grandiflora* Pers. *Tephrosia purpurea* (L.) Pers. *Trigonella foenum-graeum* Linn. *Uraria picta* Desv.
CAESALPINIACEAE
Bauhinia purpurea Linn. *Bauhinia variegata* L. *Caesalpinia crista* Linn. *Cassia absus* Linn. *Cassia angustifolia* Linn. *Cassia fistula* Linn. *Cassia occidentalis* L. *Cassia tora* Linn. *Saraca asoca* (Roxb.) de Wilde. *Tamarindus indica* Linn.
MIMOSACEAE
Acacia chundra Willd. *Acacia leucophloea* (Roxb.) Willd. *Acacia nilotica* (L.) Del subsp. *indica* (Bth.) Brenan. *Albizia lebbeck* (L.) Willd. *Prosopis cineraria* Linn.
ROSACEAE
Rosa spp.
COMBRETACEAE
Anogeissus latifolia Guill. *Terminalia arjuna* (Roxb. ex DC). Willd. and Arn. *Terminalia bellirica* (Gaertn.) Roxb. *Terminalia chebula* Retz.

MYRTACEAE
Syzygium cumini (L.) Merr. and Perry.
LECYTHIDACEAE
Careya arborea Roxb.
LYTHRACEAE
Lawsonia inermis Linn. *Woodfordia fruticosa* (Linn.) Retz.
PUNICACEAE
Punica granatum Linn.
CUCURBITACEAE
Citrullus colocynthis (Linn.) Schrad. *Luffa acutangula* (Linn.) Roem. *Luffa echinata* Roxb. *Momordica charantia* Linn. *Trichosanthes cucumerina* Linn.
APIACEAE
Anethum graveolens Linn. *Centella asiatica* (Linn.) Urb. *Cuminum cyminum* Linn. *Ferula asafoetida* Regel. *Foeniculum vulgare* Mill. *Trachyspermum ammi* (Linn.) Sprague.
ALANGIACEAE
Alangium salvifolium (L. f.) Wang.
RUBIACEAE
Cinchona spp. *Hymenodictyon orixense* (Roxb.) Wall. *Rubia cordifolia* Linn.
ASTERACEAE
Elephantopus scaber Linn. *Pluchea lanceolata* Clarke. *Sphaeranthus indicus* Linn. *Vernonia anthelmintica* (Linn.) Willd. *Vernonia cinerea* (Linn.) Less.
PLUMBAGINACEAE
Plumbago zeylanica Linn.

MYRSINACEAE
Embelia tsjeriam-cottam (R. and S.) DC.
SAPOTACEAE
Madhuca indica Muell.-Arg. *Mimusops elengi* Linn.
EBENACEAE
Diospyros melanoxylon Roxb.
OLEACEAE
Jasminum arborescens Roxb. *Jasminum multiflorum* Andr. *Nyctanthes arbortristis* Linn.
SALVADORACEAE
Salvadora persica Linn.
APOCYNACEAE
Alstonia scholaris (Linn.) R. Br. *Catharanthus roseus* (Linn.) G. Don. *Holarrhena antidysenterica* Wallich. *Nerium indicum* Mill. *Rauwolfia serpentina* (Linn.) Benth. ex Kurz.
ASCLEPIADACEAE
Calotropis procera (Aiton.) R. Br. *Leptadenia paniculata* (Retz.) W. and A.
PERIPLOCACEAE
Hemidesmus indicus (Linn.) R. Br.
LOGANIACEAE
Strychnos nux-vomica Linn.
GENTIANACEAE
Enicostema littorale (Willd.) Verdcourt. *Swertia chirayita* (Roxb. ex Flem.) Karsten.
CORDIACEAE
Cordia dichotoma Forst. f.

CONVOLVULACEAE
Argyreia nervosa (Burm. f.) Boj. *Convolvulus microphyllus* (Roth) Sieb. ex Spr. *Ipomoea digitata* Linn. *Ipomoea nil* (L.) Roth. *Ipomoea sepiaria* Koen. ex Roxb. *Merremia terpethum* (L.) Shah and Bhatt. *Datura metel* Linn. *Hyocyamus niger* Linn. *Solanum nigrum* Linn. *Solanum xanthocarpum* Burm. f. *Withania somnifera* (L.) Dunal.
SCROPHULARIACEAE
Bacopa monnieri (L.) Pennell. *Picrorrhiza kurroa* Royle ex Benth.
BIGNONIACEAE
Oroxylum indicum (L.) Venten. *Stereospermum suaveolens* (Roxb.) DC. *Tecomella undulata* (Sm.) Seem.
PEDALIACEAE
Pedalium murex Linn. *Sesamum indicum* Linn.
ACANTHACEAE
Adhatoda zeylanica Medic. *Andrographis paniculata* (Burm. f.) Wall. *Barleria prionitis* Linn. *Hygrophila auriculata* (Schum.) Heine.
VERBENACEAE
Clerodendrum multiflorum Baker. *Clerodendrum serratum* (L. f.) Gaertn. *Gmelina arborea* Roxb. *Vitex negundo* Linn.
LAMIACEAE
Lawsonia inermis Linn. *Leucas cephalotes* Spreng. *Mentha piperita* Linn. *Ocimum* sanctum, O basilicum.
PLANTAGINACEAE
Plantago major Linn.
NYCTAGINACEAE
Boerhavia diffusa Linn.
AMARANTHACEAE
Achyranthes aspera Linn. *Aerva lanata* (L.) Juss. *Celosia argentea* Linn.
POLYGONACEAE

Rheum australe Don.
ARISTOLOCHIACEAE
Aristolochia bracteolata Lam.
PIPERACEAE
Piper longum Linn.
EUPHORBIACEAE
Acalypha indica Linn. *Baliospermum montanum* (Willd.) Muell. *Euphorbia hirta* Linn. *Jatropha* curcas. *Mallotus philippensis* (Koen.) MacBr. *Phyllanthus emblica* Linn. *Phyllanthus fraternus* Webst. *Ricinus communis* Linn.
ULMACEAE
Holoptelea integrifolia (Roxb.) Planch.
MORACEAE
Ficus benghalensis Linn. *Ficus glomerata* Linn. *Ficus hispida* Linn. *Ficus religiosa* Linn.
ORCHIDACEAE
Eulophia dubia (Don.) Hochr.
ZINGIBERACEAE (SCITAMINACEAE)
Zingiber officinale Rosc. *Hedychium spicatum* Ham. ex Sm. *Curcuma longa* Linn.
HYPOXIDACEAE
Curculigo orchioides Gaertn.
DIOSCOREACEAE
Dioscorea bulbifera Linn.
LILIACEAE
Aloe indica Linn. *Allium sativum* Linn. *Asparagus racemosus* Willd var. *javanicus* Baker. *Chlorophytum borivilianum* Sant. and Fernand. *Gloriosa superba* Linn. *Urginea indica* Linn.
PANDANACEAE

Pandanus odoratissimus Lam.
TYPHACEAE
Typha angustata Bory and Chaub.
ARACEAE
Acorus calamus Linn. *Amorphophallus campanulatus* (Schott.) Engler.
CYPERACEAE
Cyperus rotundus (L.) Pers.
POACEAE
Cymbopogon martinii (Roxb.) Wats. *Desmostachya bipinnata* (Linn.) Stapf. *Saccharum officinarum* Linn.

APPENDICES

APPENDIX -I

Companies Involved in Phytopharmaceuticals Research

- Deals with name and addresses of the major pharmaceutical companies involved in R & D and manufacture of herbal drugs.
- **ANDHRA PRADESH**
- Indian Drugs and Pharmaceuticals Ltd., Research Centre. P. O. Balanagar, Hyderabad – 500073.
- **DELHI**
- Almil Pharmaceuticals Pvt. Ltd. A – 132/2 Naraina Industrial Area, Phase I. Delhi – 110028.
- Alchem International Pvt. Ltd. 240 Swami R. Tirath Nagar, Jhandewala Extension, Delhi – 110055.
- Jagson Pal and Company. 18 Bhogal Road, Jangpura. Delhi – 110014.
- Ranbaxy Laboratories Ltd. A – 1. Phase I, Okhla Industrial Area. Delhi – 110020.
- **GUJARAT**
- Alembic Chemical Works Co. Ltd. Alembic Road, Industrial Area, Vadodara – 390003, Gujarat.
- Ayurlab Pharmaceuticals Industries. K – 392, GIDC, Makarpura Industrial Estate, Vadodara – 390010, Gujarat.
- B. Tex Ointment Manufacturing Company. C – 17, Udyog Nagar, Navsari, Gujarat.
- Bharatiya Aushdhi Nirman Shala (BA(N) Dr. Vikram Sarabhai Marg, Gondal Road, Rajkot – 360004. Gujarat.
- Cadila Laboratories Pvt. Ltd. 244 Ghodasar, Maninagar, Ahmedabad, Gujarat.
- Gujarat Ayurveda University Pharmacy. Jamnagar – 361001.
- Malti-Chem Research Centre, R & D Division. (Unit of Camphor & Allied Products Ltd.) 3 GIDC Estate, Nandesari, Vadodara – 391340. Gujarat.
- Sarabhai Foundation. Vadodara, Gujarat.
- State Ayurvedic Pharmacy. Nadiad, Gujarat.
- Swami Atmanand Saraswati Sahakari Aurvedic Pharmacy, Surat.

- Unjha Pharmacy. Unjha, Gujarat.
- Vasu Pharma Pvt. Ltd. 967/4, GIDC, Makarpura Industrial Estate, Vadodara – 390010, Gujarat.

- **HARYANA**

- Indian Drugs and Pharmaceuticals Ltd. IDPL Complex, Dandahera Gurgaon Road, Gurgaon – 122001, Haryana.

- **KARNATAKA**

- Himalaya Drug Co. (P) Ltd. R & D Centre, Makali, Nelamangala. Bangalore – 562123, Karnataka.

- **MAHARASHTRA**

- Abbott Laboratories (India) Pvt. Ltd. J. B. Nagar, M. Vasanji Road, Near Vazir Glass Works, Andheri East. Mumbai – 400059.
- Alarsin Marketing (P) Ltd. A/32 Road, 3, MIDC, Andheri East. Mumbai – 400093.
- Alarsin Pharmaceuticals. 12 – K, Dubhash Road, Fort. Mumbai – 400023.
- Anglo French Drug Co. Ltd. 28 Tardeo Road, Mumbai – 400034.
- Aphali Pharmaceuticals. A – 3 Annexe, A – Z Industrial Premises, G. Kadam Marg, Mumbai – 400013.
- Atul Drug House. 85. Dr. Annie Besant Road, Worli, Mumbai – 400018.
- Ayurveda Rasashala. 25 Karve Road, Pune – 411004.
- Biddle Sawyer & Co. (India) Pvt. Ltd. 25, Dalal Street, Fort. Mumbai – 400001.
- Biological Evans Limited. Nirlon House, 1 st Floor. Dr. Annie Besant Road, Worli, Mumbai – 400018.
- Burrough's Wellcome & Co. Pvt. Ltd. 16 Bank Street, Mumbai – 400001.
- Charak Pharmaceuticals (India) Ltd. Evergreen Industrial Estate, Dr. E. Moses Road, Mumbai – 400011.
- Ciba-Geigy Research Centre. Aarey Road, Goregaon East, Mumbai – 400063.
- Cipla Ltd. 289 Bellasis Road, Bombay Central, Mumbai – 400008.
- Dulphar Interfan Ltd. 5/F Shivsagar Estate, Dr. A. B. Road, Worli, Mumbai – 400025.
- Elder Health Care Private Ltd. B – 28, Pipewala Bldg., Shahid Bhagat Singh Road, 4th Pasta Lane, Colaba, Mumbai – 400005.
- Franco-Indian Pharmaceuticals Pvt. Ltd. 20 Dr. E. Moses Road, Mumbai – 400011.
- Geoffrey Laboratories. Magnet House, Ballard Estate, Mumbai – 400038.
- Glaxo Labs (India) Ltd. Reg. Off. Dr. Annie Besant Road, Worli, Mumbai – 400025.
- Gufic Private Ltd. Subhash Road A, Vile Parle East, Mumbai – 400057.
- Hindustan Antibiotics Ltd. Pune, Maharashtra.
- Hindustan Lever Research Centre. ICT Link Road, Chakala, Andheri East, Mumbai – 400093.
- Hoechst India Ltd. Lal Bahadur Shastri Marg, Mulund, Mumbai – 400080.

- ❑ Lupin Laboratories Ltd. 159 CST Road, Kalina, Santa Cruz East, Mumbai – 400098.
- ❑ Pfizer Limited. Regd. Office. Express Towers, Nariman Point, Mumbai – 400021.
- ❑ Phyto-Pharma (Research & Development). T – 4 Neelgiri Apts. Opp. SNDT College, Karve Road, Pune, Maharashtra.
- ❑ Procter & Gamble India Ltd. Tiecicon House, Dr. E. Moses Road. Mumbai.
- ❑ Richardson Hindustan Ltd. Tiecicon House, Dr. E. Moses Road. Mumbai.
- ❑ Sandoz (India) Ltd. R & D Centre. P. O. Sandoz Baug, Kolshet Road, Thane – 400607.
- ❑ Sandu Brothers. V. N. Purav Marg, Chembur. Mumbai – 400071.
- ❑ Wockhardt Ltd. Dr. Annie Besant Road, Worli, Mumbai – 400018.
- ❑ Wyeth Laboratories Ltd. Steelcrete House, Dinshaw Wacha Road, P. O. B. 11056, Mumbai – 400020.
- ❑ Zandu Pharmaceutical Works Ltd. Gokhale Road South, Dadar, Mumbai – 400025.
- ● **TAMILNADU**
- ❑ Amrutanjan Limited Research & Development Laboratory. 42/45 Luz Church Road, Mylapore. Chennai – 60004, Tamilnadu.
- ❑ TTK Pharma Pvt. Ltd. Cathedral Road, Chennai – 600086, Tamilnadu.
- ● **UTTAR PRADESH**
- ❑ Dabur Research Foundation, Ghaziabad, U. P.
- ❑ Gurukul Kangri Pharmacy, Saharanpur District. P. O. Gurukul Kangri, Hardwar, Uttranchal.
- ❑ Harrison Laboratories, Mercantile Building, 44/101 Hospital Road. P. O. Box. 23. Kanpur – 208001.
- ❑ Himalaya Drug Co. (P) Ltd. R & D Centre. Saharanpur Road, Clement Town, Dehradun – Uttar Pradesh.
- ❑ Maharishi Ayurved Research Department, Noida Export Processing Zone, Noida, U. P.
- ● **WEST BENGAL**
- ❑ Albert David Limited, 15 Chittaranjan Avenue, Kolkatta – 700013.
- ❑ Baidyanath Ayurved Bhawan Ltd. 1 Gupta Lane, Kolkatta – 700006.
- ❑ Bengal Chemical & Pharmaceutical Works Ltd. 6 Ganesh Chander Avenue, Kolkatta – 700013.
- ❑ Dabur (Dr. S. K. Burman) Private Ltd. 142 Rasbehari Avenue, Kolkatta – 700029.
- ❑ Dey's Medical Stores (Mfg) Ltd. Research & Development Laboratory. 6/D, Neely Sengupta Sarani, Kolkatta – 700087.
- ❑ Directorate of Cinchona & Other Medicinal Plants, Govt. of West Bengal. 10/1 A, Indian Mirror Street, Kolkatta – 700013.
- ❑ Dolphin Laboratories Pvt. Ltd. 41/2 B, Sarat Bose Road, Kolkatta – 700020.
- ❑ East India Pharmaceutical Works Ltd. 6 Little Russel Street, Kolkatta.
- ❑ Himani Ltd, Kolkatta.

- Organon (India) Ltd. Himalaya House, 38 Chowringhee Road, Kolkatta – 700071.
- Standard Pharmaceuticals Ltd. 24 Park Street, Kolkatta – 700016.
- West Bengal Pharmaceutical & Phytochemical Development Corp. Ltd. ILACO House, 2nd Floor, Kolkatta – 700001.

APPENDIX-II

Major Institutes Engaged in Phytopharmaceutical and Ayurvedic Research

- Amala Cancer Research Centre (ARRC) Amala Nagar, Thrissur – 680553. Kerala.
- Arya Vaidya Sala. Malappuram District. Kottakal – 676503, Kerala.
- Arya Vaidyan Rama Varier Educational Foundation of Ayurveda (AVREF(A) 366, Trichy Road, Coimbatore – 641018. Tamilnadu.
- Bhabha Atomic Research Centre (BARC) Bioorganic Division. Trombay, Mumbai – 400085. Maharashtra.
- Bhabha Atomic Research Centre (BARC) Plant Biotechnology Section. Trombay, Mumbai – 400085. Maharashtra.
- Botanical Survey of India (BSI) Andaman and Nicobar Circle. Horticultural Road, Haddo. Port Blair – 744102.
- Botanical Survey of India (BSI) Arid Zone Circle. Jodhpur. Rajasthan.
- Botanical Survey of India (BSI) Arunachal Pradesh Circle. Sankai View, Itanagar – 791110. Arunachal Pradesh.
- Botanical Survey of India (BSI) Botanic Garden, Sibpur. Howrah – 711103, West Bengal.
- Botanical Survey of India (BSI) Central Circle. 10 Chatam Lines. Allahabad – 211001. Uttar Pradesh.
- Botanical Survey of India (BSI) Eastern Circle. Woodlands. Shillong – 793003. Meghalya.
- Botanical Survey of India (BSI) Norhtern Circle. 192. Kaulagarh Road. Dehradun – 248195. Uttar Pradesh.
- Botanical Survey of India (BSI) Sikkim Himalayan Circle. Gangtok – 737101. Sikkim.
- Botanical Survey of India (BSI) Southern Circle. P. O. Lawley Road, Tamil Nadu Agricultural University Campus. Coimbatore. 641002.
- Botanical Survey of India (BSI) Western Circle. 7, Koregaon Road, Pune – 411001. Maharashtra.
- B.V.Patel Pharmaceutical education & Research Division, Thaltej, Ahmedabad.
- Center For Advanced Pharmacological Research On Selected Traditional Remedies. Central Drug Research Institute. Chattar Manzil. P. B. 173. Lucknow – 226001. Uttar Pradesh.
- Center For Advanced Research On Standardization, Quality Control & Formulation Of Selected Traditional Remedies. (Natural Products). Punjab University, Pharmaceutical Sciences Department. Chandigarh – 160014. Punjab.
- Central Arid Zone Research Institute (CAZRI) Light Industrial Area. Jodhpur – 342003. Rajasthan.
- Central Council For Research In Ayurveda and Siddha (CCRAS) JLN Bhartiya Chikitsa Evum Homeopathy Anusandhan Bhavan, 61-65 Institutional Areas, Opp. D Block. Janakpuri. Delhi – 110058.

- Central Council For Research in Homeopathy (CCRH) JLN Bhartiya Chikitsa Evum Homeopathy Anusandhan Bhavan, 61-65 Institutional Areas, Opp. D Block. Janakpuri. Delhi – 110058.
- Central Council For Research in Unani Medicine (CCRUM) JLN Bhartiya Chikitsa Evum Homeopathy Anusandhan Bhavan, 61-65 Institutional Areas, Opp. D Block. Janakpuri. Delhi – 110058.
- Central Drug Research Institute (CDRI) Chattar Manzil Palace. Lucknow – 226001. Uttar Pradesh.
- Central Institute of Medicinal And Aromatic Plants. (CIMAP) Kukrail Picnic Spot Road. Post Bag. 1. P. O. Ram Sagar Misra Nagar. Lucknow – 226016, Uttar Pradesh.
- Central Plantation Crops Research Institute (CPCRI) Post Kudlu. Kasargod – 671124. Kerala.
- Council of Scientific And Industrial Research (CSIR) Rafi Marg. Delhi – 110001.
- Directorate of Cinchona & Other Medicinal Plants. Govt. of West Bengal. (DCOMPWB) 10/1A, Indian Mirror Street. Kolkatta – 700013. West Bengal.
- Forest Research Institute (FRI) P. O. New Forest. Dehradun – 248006. Uttranchal.
- Foundation for Revitalization of Local Health Traditions. (FRLHT) 50 – MHS Layout, 3rd Main, 2nd Stage, Anandnagar. Bangalore – 560024. Karnataka.
- Hamdard National Foundation (India). 2/3 Asaf Ali Road. Delhi – 110002.
- Homoeopathic Pharmacopoeia Laboratory (HPL) Central Government Officers Complex. Hapur Road Chungi. Ghaziabad – 201002. Uttar Pradesh.
- Indian Council Of Agricultural Research (ICAR) Krishi Anusandhan Bhavan, Pusa. Delhi – 110012.
- Indian Council of Medical Research (ICMR) Ansari Nagar. Medical Enclave. P. O. Box. 4502. Delhi – 110029.
- Indian Drugs Research Association. 516 – B, Shivajinagar. Pune – 411005. Maharashtra.
- Indian Institute of Chemical Biology (IICB) 4 Raja S. C. Mullick Road. Kolkatta – 700032. West Bengal.
- Indian Institute of Horticultural Research (IIHR) 255 Upper Palace Orchards. Bangalore – 560080. Karnataka.
- Indian Institute Of Technology (IIT) Chemistry Department. Ayurvedic Drug Development Project. Huaz Khas. Delhi – 110016.
- Institute Of Research In Indigenous System Of Medicine. Approach Road. Joginder Nagar – 176120. Himachal Pradesh.
- International Association For The Study of Traditional Asian Medicine. India. (IASTAM) Zandu Pharmaceutical Works Ltd. Gokhale Road South. Mumbai – 400025. Maharashtra.
- International Development Research Center of Canada South Asia Regional Office (IDRC – SARO) Medicinal Plants Research Network (South Asia). 17 Jor Bagh. Delhi – 110003.
- Kidwai Memorial Institute of Oncology. Indian Medicine Department. Bangalore – Karnataka.
- Lok Swasthya Parampara Samvardhan Samithi (LSPSS) P. B. 7102. Trichy Road. Ramanathapuram. Coimbatore – 641045. Tamilnadu.
- Ministry of Environment And Forests (MoEF) Paryavaran Bhawan. Central Government Office Complex, Lodi Road. Delhi – 110003.
- Ministry of Health & Family Welfare (MOHFW). Nirman Bhawan. 68 Ashoka Road. Delhi – 110011.

- Ministry of Science & Technology. Department of Biotechnology (DBT) Central Government Office Complex. Block 2, 7 th Floor. Lodi Road. Delhi – 110003.
- National Botanical Research Institute (NBRI) Rana Pratap Marg. Lucknow – 226001. Uttar Pradesh.
- National Bureau of Plant Genetic Resources (NBPGR) FIC Building, Indian Agricultural Research Institute Campus. Pusa. Delhi – 110012.
- National Chemical Laboratory (NCL) Dr. Homi Bhabha Road. Pune – 411008. Maharashtra.
- National Institute of Immunology (NII) Ayurvedic Drug Testing Project. Jawaharlal Nehru University Complex. Aruna Asaf Ali Marg. Delhi – 110067.
- Pharmacopoiel Laboratory For Indian Medicine. A Wing. 3 rd Floor. Central Government Office Building. Kamala Nehru Nagar. Ghaziabad – 201002. Uttar Pradesh.
- Publications and Information Directorate (PID) Dr. K. S. Krishnan Marg. Delhi – 110012.
- Regional Research Laboratory. Bhubaneshwar (RRL- Bhubaneshwar). Sachivalya Marg. Bhubaneshwar – 751013. Orissa.
- Regional Research Laboratory. Jammu (RRL – Jammu). Canal Road. Jammu Tawi – 180001. Jammu & Kashmir.
- Regional Research Laboratory. Jammu (RRL – Jammu). Extension Centre. Palampur. Himachal Pradesh.
- Regional Research Laboratory. Jammu (RRL – Jammu). Field Research Station. Experimental Farm. Jammu Cantonment. Chatha. Jammu & Kashmir.
- Regional Research Laboratory. Jorhat (RRL – Jorhat). Branch Laboratory. Naharlagun. P. O. Itanagar – 791110. Arunachal Pradesh.
- Regional Research Laboratory. Jorhat (RRL – Jorhat). Jorhat – 785006. Assam.
- Regional Research Laboratory. Thiruvananthapuram (RRL – Thiruvananthapuram). P. O. Industrial Estate. Pappanamcode. Thiruvananthapuram – 695019. Kerala.
- Shri Bapalal Vaidhya Botanical Research Centre, S.G.U. Surat.
- Tamilnadu Government Cinchona Department. Nilgiris P. Box. 06. Udhagamandalam – 643001. Tamilnadu.
- Tibetan Medical & Astro Institute (MEN – TSEE – KHANG) Khara Danda Road. Kangra District. Dharamsala – 176215. Himachal Pradesh.
- Tropical Botanic Graden & Research Institute (TBGRI) Karimancode. Pacha – Palode. P. O. Thiruvananthapuram – 692562. Kerala.
- Tropical Forest Research Institute. (TFRI) Mandla Road. Jabalpur – 482001. Madhya Pradesh.
- United Nations Educational Scientific & Cultural Organization (UNESCO) Regional Office Of Science & Technology For South & Central Asia. 8. Poorvi Marg. Vasant Vihar. Delhi – 110057.
- Voluntary Health Association of India (VHAI) Tong Swasthya Bhawan, 40 Qutab Institutional Areas. South of IIT. Delhi – 110016.
- World Health Organization. South East Asia Regional Office. (WHO – SEARO) Indrapastha Estate, Mahatma Gandhi Road. Delhi – 110002.

APPENDIX-III

Suppliers of Herbal Extracts and Phytochemicals in India

- Alchem International Pvt. Ltd., 240, Jhandewalan Extension, New Delhi – 110055 – Phytochemicals.
- Alembic Chemical Works. Baroda. Gujarat – Extracts.
- Alkaloids Corporation. 8, Bentick Street, Kolkatta – 700001 – Phytochemicals.
- Amsar Private Ltd.47 Laxmibai Nagar Industrial Estate. Fort. Indore – 452006 – Extracts, Phytochemicals and Essential Oils.
- Ansar Drugs Laboratories, Salabbatpura, Moti Begumwadi, Surat – 395002 – Extracts.
- Auro Impex Pvt. Ltd., 8 C-1-4936, Dehgam Road, Industries Township, Vapi – 396195 – Phytochemicals.
- Bengal Chemicals & Pharmaceuticals Ltd. 153. Dharamtala Street. Kolkatta – 700013 – Extracts.
- Bengal Chemicals & Pharmaceuticals Ltd. 164, Maniktala Main Road, Kolkatta – 700054 – Extracts.
- Bicon India Pvt. Ltd. 20th KM Hosur Road, Hebbagodi 562158, Bangalore District – Papain.
- Biological Evans Ltd., C-1-4936, Dehgam Road, Industries Township, Vapi – 396195 – Phytochemicals.
- Bombay Extractions Pvt. Ltd. Daya Mandir, 1st Floor, 123-25, Mumbadevi Road, Mumbai – 400003 – Castor Oil.
- Chemical, Industrial & Pharmaceuticals Laboratories Ltd. Vikhroli, Mumbai – 400079 – Phytochemicals.
- Chemiloids, 40-45, 10B, Brindavan Colony, Labbipet, Vijaywada 510010 – Extracts, Phytochemicals and Essential Oils.
- CIBA –Geigy of India Ltd. Bhandup, Mumbai – 400078 – Phytochemicals.
- CIMAP, CSIR Institution. Lucknow – 226016 – Essential Oils.
- CIPLA Research Centre & Factory, Vigonagar. P & T Office, Bangalore – Phytochemicals.
- Drug Research Laboratory (Farm and Factories J & K), Jammu Tawi – 180001 – Extracts and Phytochemicals.
- Enzo Chem Laboratories Pvt. Ltd. Maharashtra – Papain.
- Glaxo Laboratories Pvt. Ltd. Dr. Annie Besant Road, Worli, Mumbai – 400018 – Phytochemicals.
- Government Opium and Alkaloid Works, Ghaziapur (U. P) – Opium alkaloids.
- Government Quinine Factory, Anamallai, Tamilnadu – Quinine Salts.
- Herbochem, 38. Technocrats Industrial Estate. Balanagar. Hyderabad – 500037 – Herbal Extracts.
- Indo German Alkaloids, Mahakali Caves Road, Andheri (East), Mumbai – 400093 – Phytochemicals.
- Jayant Oil Mills, 13 Sitalwadi, Mazgaon, Mumbai – Castor oil.
- Kisalaya Pharmaceuticals Pvt. Ltd. Plot No. 548, Sector III, Industrial Area, Pithampur District, Dhar (M.P) – Tannic Acid.
- Kothari Phytochemicals International, 766, Anna Nagar, Madurai – 625020 – Phytochemicals.
- Kulu Aromatics, Shamshi – 175126. District Kullu, Himachal Pradesh – Essential Oils.

- Kumaon Chemical Products, Village Shivalalpur. P. O. Ramnagar – 244715, Nainital – Phytochemicals and Ginger Oil.
- Liberty Oil Mills Pvt Ltd., 302. Dalamal House, 206 Nariman Point, Mumbai – 400021 – Castor Oil.
- Mehta Pharmaceuticals Pvt. Ltd. G – T Road, Chheharta. Amritsar 143105 – Brucine Sulphate, Berberine Hydrochloride, Podophyllum Resin BP/USP, Sentonin IP/JP, Strychnine, Calcium sennosides A +B, Xanthotoxin (USP), Methoxsalen, Valerian extract and Herbal extracts.
- New India Agro Chemical Industries. 4013, Yawai Road. Bhusawal – Phytochemicals.
- Organochem Laboratories, Near Janata Vidyalaya, Yeola District, Nasik – Phytochemicals.
- Polybond Chemicals, 4, Bhaktinagar Station Plot, Rajkot – 360002 – Papain.
- Rathi Papains Pvt. Ltd. 75-76 A, Mittal Court, Nariman Point, Mumbai – 400021 – Papain.
- Regional Research Laboratory, Jammu Tawi – Phytochemicals.
- Sandoz India Ltd. Sandoz House, Dr. Annie Besant Road, Worli, Mumbai – 400018 – Phytochemicals.
- Shashi Phytochemicals Industry, 1. Old Industrial Area. Alwar – Phytochemicals.
- Sheeba Laboratories Pvt. Ltd., B-151. Avas Vikas Colony, Delhi Road, Saharampur – 247001 – Phytochemicals.
- Smith Stainstreet Pharmaceuticals Ltd. 18, Convent Road, Kolkatta – 700014 – Phytochemicals.
- Standard Essential Oil Distillers, 84/113. Carvalongar, Kanpur – 208003 – Essential oils.
- True Food Corporation, 17, Kamer Building, 38, Cawasji Patel Street, Mumbai – 400023 – Papain.
- Uma Ayurveda Bhawan Pvt. Ltd. Kasganj, Uttar Pradesh – 207123 – Extracts, Phytochemicals, Bhasmas.

APPENDIX-IV

World wide Traders of Natural Products

BELGIUM

- Codidex Pharma SPRL, Rue Josse-Impems, 1030 Brussels, Belgium. Tel : 32-02-2415324. Fax : 21662993.
- Du Pont De Nemours (Belgium). 100, Rue De La Fusee, B-1130, Bruxelles. Belgium. Tel : 32-02-7242611. Fax : 32-6210460.
- Hybritech Europe S. A. 12, All Des Noisetiers, S. A. B-4900 Angleur, Belgium. Tel : 32-41677000. Fax : 32-676210.
- PARC Scientifique, Rue Du Bosquet 7, B-1348 Louvain-La-Neuve, Belgium. Tel : 0032-10-455257. Fax : 0032-10-456076/454934.
- Sofarex N. V. Van Varenberghstraat 49, B-2600, Berchem. Antwerp, Belgium. Tel : 32-32189032. Fax : 32-3189955.
- Somejant Sa. Rue De Boetendael 147. B-1190, Bruxelles, Belgium. Fax : 32-23453806.
- Thissen S. A. Laboratories. 4-6 Rue De La Papyree. B-1420. Briane Ualeud, Belgium. Tel : 32-23861211. Fax : 32-3851782.

FRANCE

- Docks Des Alcools SA. 57 Rue De Villiers, F – 92200. Neuilly Sur Seine, France. Tel : 33-147572420.

GREECE

- ❑ Vioergex V. Salatas Sons Ltd. 35 Deligiorgi St., GR-10437, Athens, Greece. Tel : 30-01-5237484, 5242271.

GERMANY

- ❑ Homviora Arznei Hagedorn Gmbh. Arabellastrasse 5, D-8000. Munchen 81, Germany. Tel : 49-089-92322800.
- ❑ Introplant Tropenpflanzen. Trottstrasse 16, D-350. Kassel, Germany. Tel : 49-0561-300013.
- ❑ Pfannenschmidt. P. O. Box 20224. D-2000. Hamburg 54. Germany. Tel : 49-0405531057. Fax : 49-0405536414.
- ❑ Varhaelen GMBH. Muelheimmer Str. 176. W-4100. Duisburg. Germany. Tel : 49-0203-355005. Fax : 49-0203-355006.

ITALY

- ❑ Ely Lilly Italia SPA. Via Gmsci. 733. I – 50019 Sesto Florentino (Fi), Italy. Tel : 39-5542130.
- ❑ Istituto Gentili SPA. Via Mazzini. 112. I-56100 Pisa. Italy. Tel : 39-50501980.
- ❑ Sclavo SPA. Via Fiorentina, 1-I-53100 Siena, Italy. Tel : 39-5772931111.

PORTUGAL

- ❑ Aquario Commercio De Electronica. Rue De Algeria 93-A. 4000 Porto Portugal. Tel : 02-323381,318817. Fax : 02-2001379.

RUSSIA

- ❑ Medexport. Import Dept. 31, Korp. 2. Ul Kakhovka. Moscow 113461, Russia. Tel : 07-1210154.

SPAIN

- ❑ Borrasosa SL C/Locom. 5. Cabezo de Torres. E-30110 Murcia. Spain. Tel : 34-05-4359669.
- ❑ Industrias La Locomotora SL. C/Locom. 5, Cabezo De Torres. E-30110. Murcia. Spain. Tel : 34-68831025. Fax : 34-68832017.
- ❑ Laboratorio de Applicationes. Calle Lope de Ruedo 46. E-30220. Madrid. Spain. Tel : 34-01-57440342. Fax : 34-01-5736537.

KUWAIT

- ❑ Gulf Delta Corp. P. O. Box. 252. Safat 13003, Kuwait. Tel : 965-4814499. Fax : 965-4837817.

POLAND

- ❑ Rolimpex. P. O. Box 364. PL-00950. Warszawa, Poland. Tel : 48-301000 / 300636. Fax : 48-301867.

SWITZERLAND

- ❑ Equilibrium SA. 8, Route De Buchillon, Ch-1162. Saint Prex, Switzerland. Tel : 41-021-8062245. Fax : 41-021-8062109.

SYRIA

- ❑ Bechara Yordan Obegi. PO Box. 343. Damascus, Syria. Tel : 17693.

UNITED KINGDOM (UK)

- ❑ Anard Mount Ltd. West Africa House, Ashbourne R. CB – London W5 3QP, England. Tel : 44-819915150. Fax : 44-819915001.
- ❑ Bush Beach Ltd. Stanley Green Ltd. GB – Cheadle Hu. Cheadle SK8 6RN, England. Tel : 44-61/4858231. Fax : 44-61/4856445.

- Mr. A. A. Spencer. 69 Pine Grove Brookmans Park. BG – Hatfield AL9 7BL, England. Tel : 44-707/55354. Fax : 44-1/4409928.

OMAN

- United National Commercial Co. P. O. Box. 4428, Ruwi, Oman. Tel : 706670 / 796701.

SAUDI ARABIA

- Bafarat Spices and Herbs Shops. P. O. Box. 11652. Jeddah 21463, Saudi Arabia. Tel : 966-6421058. Fax : 966-6433379.
- Mootah Medical Co. P. O. Box. 17561. Jeddah 21494, Saudi Arabia. Tel : 966-026400196 / 6400918.
- Mobarak H Al Dosari. P. O. Box. No. 59462. Riyadh 11532. Saudi Arabia. Fax : 2332585.

BAHRAIN

- Baharain Pharmacy & Gen. Store. P. O. Box. 56, Manama, Bahrain. Tel : 973-253491.

ARGENTINA

- Michans Y Roy Ltd. Florida 737, Piso 1, Off. 1005 Buenos Aires, Argentina. Tel : 54-01-322-1322.

CANADA

- Flora Distributors Ltd. 7400 Fraser Park Drive, Burnaby. BC V5 B9, Canada. Tel : 697-4366000. Fax : 604-4366050.
- Wing Hing Co. Ltd. 8823 E Cordova St. Vancouver. BC V6A 1M5. Canada. Telex : 04-352848.

UNITED STATES OF AMERICA (USA)

- Botanicals International. 2550 El Presidio Street. Long Beach CA 90810. USA. Tel : 310-637-9566. Fax : 310-637-3644.
- Cyclo Products Inc. P. O. Box. 01557. Los Angeles. CA 90001. USA. Tel : 213-582-6411. Fax : 213-582-8038.
- F. H. Taussig Inc. 111 Brook St. Scarsdale, NY 10583. USA. Tel : 914-472-6464. Fax : 914-472-1846.
- Foreign Domestic Chemicals 95 Chestnut Ridge Road. Montvale NJ 07645. USA. Tel : 201-307-3333. Fax : 201-307-3387.
- G. D. Searle. 5200 Old Orchard Rd. Skokie. IL 60077. USA. Tel : 708-470-3028. Fax : 708-967-2099.
- Golomback Morris J. Inc. 960-Franklin Ave. Brooklyn. NY 11225. USA. Tel : 718-284-3505. Fax : 718-693-1941.
- Hauser Chemical Research Inc. 4750 Nautilus Court. S. Boulder. 80301. USA. Tel : 303-530-4750. Fax : 303-530-7083.
- Herbarium Inc. 11016 152nd Ave. Kenosha WI 53142. USA. Tel : 414-857-2373. Fax : 718-693-1941.
- Mayway Corporation. 1338 Cypress St. Mandela Pkwy. Oakland. CA 94607. USA. Tel : 510-208-3113. Fax : 510-208-3069.
- Olfactory Corporation. PO Box. 21620. Oxnard. CA 93034. USA. Tel : 805-644-8955.
- Sunrider International. 3111 Lomita BL Vd. Torrance. CA. 90505. USA. Tel : 310-534-4786.
- The Lebermuth Co. P. O. Box. 4103. South Bend. IN 46634. USA. Tel : 219-259-7000. Fax : 219-258-7450.
- Whole Herb Co. P. O. Box. 1085. Mill Valley. CA 94942. USA. Tel : 415-383-6485. Fax : 415-383-1747.

AUSTRALIA

- Herbimex GPO Box 1514. Brisbane QLD 4001, Australia. Tel : 61-07-2854454.

CHILE

- Laboratorio Vitafarma Ltd. PO Box 51130. Santiago, Chile. Tel : 56-02-2742332. Fax : 56-02-2742407.

JAPAN

- Alps Pharmacueticals Ind. Co. Ltd. USUJI – Koraibashi Bldg, 4-7 Koraibashi 2-Chome, Osaka 541, Japan. Tel : 81-06-201-4561. Fax : 81-06-223-8876.
- Crew Corp. 10-9-606, Uehommachi. 6-Chome. Tennoji-Ku, Osaka 543, Japan. Tel : 81-06-733-2118. Fax : 81-06-773-1813.
- Dainan Boeki Kaishi Ltd. 3-3, Minami-Kyuhoji-Machi. 3-Chome, Chuo-Ku, Osaka 541, Japan. Tel : 81-06-251-1191. Fax : 81-06-251-1192.
- Fukunda Ryu Co. Ltd. 5-11 Nishitemma 1-Chome. Kita-Ku, Osaka 530, Japan. Tel : 81-06-364-5861. Fax : 81-06-364-6562.
- Hino Pharmaceutical C. Ltd. 3-15, Koshomachi 2-Chome. Chuo-Ku, Osaka 541, Japan. Tel : 81-06-231-5847. Fax : 81-06-231-7309.
- Hip Shing Tai Co. (Japan) Ltd. PO Box 620, Kobe Port, Kobe 650, Japan. Tel : 81-078-391-2191.
- Ichimaru Co. Ltd. J. Bldg. 3-7, Cushimimachi, 2-Chome, Bhuo-Ku, Osaka 541, Japan. Tel : 81-06-2010612. Fax : 81-06-201-0617.
- Korishita Jintan Co. Ltd. 1-30, Tamatsukuri 1-Chome.Chuo-Ku, Osaka 540, Japan. Tel : 81-06-761-1133. Fax : 81-06-768-1661.
- Koshiro Co. Ltd. 5-8 Doshomachi 2-Chome. Chuo-Ku, Osaka 541, Japan. Tel : 81-06-231-1803. Fax : 81-06-227-0187.
- Koyaku Company Limited. 13-1 Shimosone Shinmachi. Kokuram-Ku, Kitakyushu 80002, Japan. Tel : 81-093-471-1981. Fax : 81-471-1862.
- Manage Develop. Fukunaga Co. Ltd. 457-8, Tonochara. Chikushino City, 818. Japan. Tel : 81-092-922-2028. Fax : 81-092-924-4710.

PHILIPPINES

- Pharma Industries Inc. PO Box 604, Manila, Philippines. Tel : 53-885-311.

MALAYSIA

- Heron Products (M) Sdn. Bhd. 10-A JL, Jejaka 7, T. Mal Cheras. 55100, Kaula Lumpur. Malaysia. Tel : 60-3-9858552. Fax : 60-3-9858366.
- Natures Herbs Sdn. Bhd. 62, 1/F Jalan SS 2/66. 47300 Petaling. Jaya, Selangor, Malaysia. Tel : 60-3-7765887. Fax : 60-3-7765887.
- Voon Ng Tong Trading Co. Bhd. 489 Jalan Sungei Rambai 14000 Bukit Mertajam, Malaysia. Tel : 60-04-511533.
- Nature's Sunshine Products. 95A, Jalan Jejaka Sembilan. 55100 Kuala Lumpur, Malaysia. Tel : 60-03-9852722. Fax : 60-03-9856231.
- UHA Marketing (M) Sdn. Bhd. 8 JL Mega Mend. 5/M Old Klang. 58200 Kuala Lumpur, Malaysia. Tel : 60-3-7839536. Fax : 60-3-7817353.
- Weng Aun Thye. 258 Lebuh Pantai. 10300 Penang, Malaysia. Tel : 60-04-612310 / 622200.

SOUTH KOREA

- Dooley International Corp. CPO Box 10696. Seoul, South Korea. Tel : 82-02-2520741, 2355713. Fax : 82-02-2360040.

- Pharmaton-Korea Co. Ltd. CPO Box. 2533, Seol, South Korea. Tel : 82-02-755-3788. Fax : 82-02-7546732.

EGYPT

- Ankram Company. 30, Abdel Raheim Sabri Street. Dokki, Cairo, Egypt. Tel : 20-709093.
- N. I. Ibrahim Company (Flavogypt). 8, Falaki Street, Alexandria, Egypt. Tel : 20-3-4825064. Fax : 20-3-4833923.

APPENDIX-V

Pratinidhi Dravya - Substitute Drugs used :—

	ORIGINAL DRUG		SUBSTITUTE DRUG	
Sr. #	**SANSKRIT NAME**	**BOTANICAL NAME**	**SANSKRIT NAME**	**BOTANICAL NAME**
01	Chitrak	*Plumbago zeylanica*	Danti	*Baliospermum montanum*
02	Dhanyaghas	*Fagonia cretica*	Pavasak	*Alhagi psuedalhagi*
03	Tagar	*Valeriana wallichii*	Kustha	*Saucerea lappa*
04	Murva	*Clematis gouriana*	Manjistha	*Rubia cordifolia*
05	Bakul	*Mimusops elengi*	Nilkamal	*Nelumbo nucifera*
06	Nilkamal	*Nelumbo nucifera*	Kumudpushpa	*Nymphaea stellata*
07	Chameli pushpa	*Jasminum officinalis*	Laving	*Syzygium aromaticum*
08	Arkakshir	*Calotropis procera*	Arkapatra	*Calotropis procera*
09	Pushakarmool	*Inula racemosa*	Kushta	*Saucerea lappa*
10	Snuhi	*Euphorbia neriifolia*	Kustha	*Saucerea lappa*
11	Chavya	*Piper cubeba*	Pipali	*Piper longum*
12	Daru haridra	*Berberis aristata*	Haridra	*Curcuma longa*
13	Bharangi	*Clerodendrum serratum*	Talispatra	*Taxus baccata*
14	Yastimadhu	*Glycyrrhiza glabra*	Dhatakipushpa	*Woodfordia fruticosa*
15	Rajavriksha	*Cassia fistula*	Chukra	*Rumex vesicarius*
16	Draksha	*Vitis vinifera*	Gambhariphal	*Gmelina arborea*

Sourse : Status, cultivation and conservation of Medicinal Plants, Report, Anonymous, 2000.

17	Gambhari	*Gmelina arborea*	Madhukapushpa	*Madhuca indica*
18	Chinikabab	*Piper cubeba*	Chamelipushpa	*Jasminum officinale*
19	Karpur	*Cinnamomum camphora*	Nagarmusta	*Cyperus rotundus*
20	Kesar	*Crocus sativus*	Kusumphool	*Carthamus tinctorius*
21	Swetachandan	*Santalum album*	Karpur	*Cinnamomum camphora*
22	Swetachandan	*Santalum album*	Raktachandan	*Pterocarpus santalinus*
23	Raktachandan	*Pterocarpus santalinus*	Ushir	*Vetiveria zizinoides*
24	Haritaka	*Terminalia chebula*	Amalki	*Emblica officinalis*
25	Ativish	*Aconitum ferox*	Nagarmustak	*Cyperus rotundus*
26	Nagkesar	*Messua ferea*	Kamal kesar	*Nelumbo nucifera*
27	Bhallatak	*Semicarpus anacardium*	Chitraka	*Plumbago zeylanica*
28	Danti	*Baliospermum montanum*	Chitraka	*Plumbago zeylanica*
29	Meda	*Polygonum glabrum*	Shatavari	*Asparagus racemosus*
30	Mahameda	*Polygonum verticillatum*	Shatavari	*Asparagus racemosus*
31	Jivaka	*Microstylis wallichii*	Vidarikand	*Pueraria tuberosa*
32	Rhushabhak	*Microstylis muscifera*	Vidarikund	*Pueraria tuberosa*
33	Kakoli	*Rosa procera*	Ashwagandha	*Withania somnifera*
34	Kshirkakoli	*Lilium polyphyllum*	Ashwagandha	*Withania somnifera*
35	Ruddhi	*Habenaria intermedia*	Varahikand	*Dioscorea bulbifera*
36	Vruddhi	*Habernaria spp.*	Varahikand	*Dioscorea bulbifera*

APPENDIX-VI

Adulterants used :—

Sr. #	NAME OF THE DRUG	PLANTS AND OTHER MATERIAL USED FOR ADULTERATION/ ADULTERANTS
1	Arjun chhal (Bark) (White sadad) *Terminalia arjuna*.	Baheda, Krishna arjun, Harde, Deshi Almond and bark of other species.
2	Ashok chhal (Bark of *Saraca asoca*).	Shal, Trayman, Asopalav (*Polyalthia longifolia*) and Kanchar Chhal (Bauhinia spp).
3	Guggal gum (*Commiphora wightii*)	Balsam, Usak Loban, Hirabol, Bhammarchhal, (Hymenodictyam excelsum) Shallaki (*Boswellia serrata*) and other gum. Sand and soil are also be mixed.
4	Hing (*Ferula asafoetida*)	Resin with smell, painted gum, gum of bawal (*Acacia*), brown soil, corn flour.
5	Kesar	Nyctanthus spp painted corn style, *Calendula officinalis*, *Carthamus tinctorius*. Stamen and other flowers can be mixed.
6	Ativish	Vakhmo and bulb of *cryptocoryne retrospiralis*,
7	Kasturi	Animal blood, liver pieces, dry peas, wheat – barley mixture. Also Amretta seed, Angelia root, Guaria grandiflora bark etc. Plants that give smell like Kasturi, Nabhi of other animals is also used as Kasturinabhi.
8	Jayphal (*Myristica fragrans*)	Other fruits without oil e.g; *Myristica malabarica* are pushed in.
9	Laving (*Piper longum*)	Original laving without oil, which gives less smell.
10	Elaichi	Original Elaichi without oil.
11	Taj (*Cinnamomum tamala*)	Bark of other plants and original Taj without oil.
12	Brahmi (*Centella asiatica*)	Undarkani's panchang (*Merremia emarginata* Whole plant).
13	Vidari kand (*Pueraria tuberosa*)	Cycas-Kangutad's root pieces.
14	Ganthoda (*Piper root*)	Branches and pieces of other plants like different species of Piper.
15	Shal parni	*Alysicarpus tetragonolobus* (Samervo) and other genus.
16	Patol (*Trichosanthes cucumerina*)	Panchang of Karela and other cucurbitaceous climbers (*Momordica charantia*).

17	Vanskapoor	Tungakehari (Curcuma angustifolia), root pieces and synthetic vanskapoor.
18	Lindi piper (Piper longum)	Big thick fruits of Piper spp.
19	Masparni (jangli adad) (Phaseolus aureus)	Climbers of magamathi (Rhynchosia minima)
20	Kapilo (Mallotus phillippensis)	Dust of brick, red soil, colour etc.
21	Nagkesar	Stamen of any other plants and undeveloped Puspkalika of Surpunakh (Ochrocarpus longifolia), Seeds of Mehndi. (Lawsonia spp).
22	Kasth-uplet	Plant of tulsiphool (Ocimum spp), Salvia lanata and Costus speciosus. Also Puskarmool is useful.
23	Swet chandan (Santalum album)	Pieces of innerwood and pith of other plants.
24	Mochras	Gum of simlo, red soil, chhal (bark) of other plants.
25	Kakdasingi	Round, oval, flat formations on plants made by insects, i. e. insect galls.
26	Tamalpatra (Cinnamomum tamala)	Leaves of Taj, Laving and Cinnamomum spp.
27	Rasna (Pluchea lanceolata)	Damvel, Ishwari, Kulijan, Puskarmool, Vaisuri, Kaknuj, Viscum articulatum.
28	Bharangimool (Clerodendrum multiflorum)	Pieces of other plant branches. Bark of Picrorrhiza quassioides.

APPENDIX - VII

Plants Restricted for Export

PLEASE REFER ZEROX COPY ENCLOSED AND PASTE HERE NEED FOR GOOD AGRICULTURAL PRACTICES AS A MODERN TOOL FOR AYURVEDIC PRACTICES

- Following are the pre-requisite for the farmer interested in cultivation of medicinal plants.
- Knowledge about good agricultural practice for good cultivation obtained through State Agriculture Universities IRRI. Institute of Council of Scientific & Industrial Research.
- Availablity of authentic seeds/cuttings/planting material for plantation at a reasonable rate through state wise special agencies.
- Farmers should be encouraged by State Govt. and Central Govt. through low cost medicinal crop insurance. Help should be extended for soil testing, water quality testing and diseases management and menure management through concerned faculties or agencies. Farmers may be subsidies for preparing borewell, check dams and such other water management recharge & conservation schemes.

- Primary processing and value addition methods be developed, standardized and made available farmers as Lab to Land technology transfer projects promotion of desigining and supply of solar dryers could be boon the farmers.
- Drying of Herbs, leaves, Seeds, Flowers, Roots. This is one of the major problems and fungus and insects infect mainly partly dried material. Good, easy drying and economic drying process for roots, fruits, flowers, stem, leaves, barks should be developed by scientist and government by involving efficient engineering technocrats to come out with cheaper efficient dryers specially using solar energy. Drying in rainy season used to be a problem. This has to be over scientifically and at economic rate.
- Storage of dry material. This is another area where farmers need help dry material in rainy season absorbs moisture and turn wet leading to fungal infection and insects development. Scientist should suggest cheapest way of storage of dry herbs in perfect and scientific manner. Wet herbs, collected for drying also need special attention for storage till these are dried.
- Quality awareness where farmer should be aware mainly on three aspects. (1). Proper harvesting. (2). Drying of harvested material and (C) Proper marketing of finished products.
- Presently the farmers are not getting proper price. Wholesale traders offer meagre price only. Wholesale traders also face fear of market price and uncertainity of storage period till product is sold. They have to continuously look after stored goods and throw away infected material. This causes rise in price on part of manufactures. A chain has to be developed from farmer to trader to manufacturer so that all can get benefit of price with quality material.

Guidelines for Good Agricultural Practices (G.A.P) of Medicinal and Aromatic Plants

- General part includes scope, proper environmental conditions, availability of seeds and propagation material, cultivation, soil and fertilization, proper irrigation facilities, harvest, primary processing, packaging, storage and transport, equipment, personnel and facilities, documentation, education and quality assurance.

Quality Control of Herbal Materials

- In view of acceptance of herbal medicament world over and in the larger interest of phenomenol growth of herbal industries, it is the need the of time to develop and implement Q. C measures.
- The mordern techniques of Q.C Gas Chromatrography (GC), Gas Liquid Chromatorgraphy (GLC), Gas Solid Chromatrography (GSC), High Pressure Liquid Chromatorgraphy (HPLC), High Performance Thin Layer Chromatography (HPTLC), UV and IR Spectrophotometre , Atomic Absorption Spectrophotometere.

Sampling

- Due to very specific properties and peculiarities of materials while taking samples following procedures should be observed.
- Strict inspection of each container with reference to claims, labels etc.
- If containers are more select the samples from top, middle and bottom of the container for random testing.
- Inspect the same for organo-leptic characteristics, presence of foreign matter, sign of decay if any, presence of fungus, insects etc.
- Average sample must be tested for sieve test, impurities, moisture and ash content, level of active ingredients where possible.
- Macroscopic and microscopic examinations must be carried out.

- The sample size recommended for plants are as follows:-(1). Roots, rhizomes and bark – sample size 500 g. (2). Leaves, Flowers, Fruits and Seeds – 250 g. (3). Cut medicinal plant material – 50 g.

Basic Criteria

- Temperature should be expressed in degree celcius.
- Test should be conducted at room temperature i.e. 15 – 25 ^{O} C.
- Glassware to be used should be of good quality and calibrated. Also water bath should be with boiling water and solutions must be prepared in distilled water.
- Solubility, proper storage, utilization well closed containers, protection from sunlight, humidity control, cut size of plant materials etc should be followed strictly.
- Powder's fineness should be as per WHO guidelines as follows. (1). Coarse: all particles will pass through 2000-sieve size. (2). Moderately coarse: 710 – sieve size. (3). Moderately Fine particles – 355 sieve size. (4). Fine particles through 180 sieve size. (5). Very Fine particles through 125 sieve size.
- Sieve numbers mentioned above are as per conformations to ISO standard 565, 1990.

Macrosopic Examination

- Visual check is simple and quick. Confirmation of size, colour, odour, taste etc. Many suppliers are active to provide substitute or adulterants and can easily misguide users. It is expected to substantiate findings by microscopic examinations.

Microscopic Examination

- Dried parts should be softened; hard parts should be soaked in water.
- For achieving transparent leaves boil them on slides. For thicker leaves cut them in pieces and treat with Chloral hydrate. To remove thick epidermal layer treat with glycerol or ethanol.
- Sections should be Transverse Section or Longitudinal Section by razor blade or microtome.
- To achieve of T. S. or L. S. (by dissolving starch grains, plastids, fats, oilseeds) the reagents like Chloral hydrate and Lactochloral, Lactophenol, Sodium hypochlorite, Light Petroleum reagents should be used.
- For histochemical detection of cell wall and its contents Iodine, Sulphuric Acid, Phloroglucinol, HCL, Sudan Red, Chinese ink, Ferric Chloride etc are to be used.

Some Important Guidelines for Q.A. of Medicinal Plants

- Some of the important determinations to be performed are as follows.
- Ash.

- Extractable matter.
- Water and volatile matter.
- Volatile oil.
- Bitterness value.
- Haemolytic activity.
- Pesticide residues.
- Arsenic and heavy metals.
- Microorganisms.
- Radioactive contamination.

Pesticide Residues

- Agricultural practices have been generating huge amount of pesticide residues. Some are with long residual action e.g; Chlorinated Hydrocarbons and Carbophenothion.

Determination of Arsenic and Heavy Metals

- Environmental pollution and traces of pesticides are among many causes to contaminate plant materials with arsenic and heavy metals world over. Recommended procedures are followed to determine limit test for arsenic and limit test for cadmium and lead.

Limit of Microbial Contamination in Herbal Material

- The naturally inherent microbial load of crude plant material maximum 10^4 per g and for mould propagules is maximum 10^5 per g.
- The microbial load of pretreated plant material for aerobic bacteria is maximum 10^7 per g; for , yeast and moulds is maximum 10^4 per g and for E. coli is maximum 10^2 per g and other enterobacteria maximum 10^4 per g.
- For other plant material of internal use aerobic bacteria maximum 10^5 per gm, yeast and moulds maximum 10^3 per gm, E. coli maximum 10^2 per gm and other enterobacteria maximum 10^3 per gm.

Recent Trends of Quality Assurance

- The use of chromatographic techniques and marker compounds to standardize botanical preparation have limitations. DNA based molecular markers (PCR Technique) have utility in the authentication of plant species of medicinal values. The new pharmacognosy includes all aspects of drug development and discovery where biotechnology driven application play an important role. Current focus on chemotype driven fingerprinting and related techniques requires integration with genotype driven molecular technique so that maximum characterization of botanical materials is possible. Also this is very useful to discard substitutes widely used instead of genuine plant material. Extensive research on DNA based molecular markers is in progress in many research institutes through out world particularly in China. In India several agricultural universities and research institutions are involved and are following DNA-based techniques in genotyping of medicinal plants. It is an open field for researchers to intigrate molecular techniques and analytical tools that will lead to the development of comprehensive system of botanical characterization that can be conveniently applied to industry for quality control of herbal materials.
- SOURCE – Current Science. Vol. **87.** No. **2.** July 2004.

SUGGESTED READING AND REFERENCE CITATION

1. Charaksamhita. Sushrutsamhita. Bhav Prakash. Arya Bhisak. Sarangdharsamhita. Shree Dhanvantri Nighuntu.
2. Ratnavali. Ratnamala. Madhav-krut Dravyavali.
3. Medicinal plants by Dr. S.K. Jain. 1968. National Book Trust. New Delhi.
4. Selected Indian Medicinal plants- Chemexcil Publication. 1992. SPIC Foundation. Madras.
5. Indian Medicinal Plants (Vol I-12). Late Kirtikar, K. R. and B. D. Basu. 1980. Revised and Enlarged by Blatter, Caius and Mahaskar. Reprinted by M/s. Bishen Singh Mahendra Pal Singh, Dehradun.
6. 'Kutchni Vanaspati' By Jaikrishna Indraji Thaker. Pravin Pustakalay. Rajkot.
7. Vanaspatishastra By Jaikrishna Indraji Thaker. Pravin Pustakalay. Rajkot.
8. Nighantu (I and II) By Late Acharya Bapalal Vaidya. 1999. Gujarat Pustakalaya Sahayak Sahakari Mandal Ltd. Vadodara.
9. Pharmacopoeial Standards of Indian Herbal Plants- C. R. Karnick.
10. Indian Medicinal Plants Used in Ayurvedic Preparations- A. C. Dey. 1980. Bishen Singh Mahendra Pal Singh, Dehradun.
11. Herbs That Heal- H. K. Bakhru. 1995. Orient Paperbacks, New Delhi.
12. Medicinal Plants of India with Special Reference to Ayurveda- C. K. N. Nair and N. Mohanan. 1998. Nag Publishers. New Delhi.
13. Indigenous Drugs of India- R. N. Chopra. 1962. Tropical School of Medicine, Kolkatta.
14. Wealth of India. (A to Z). CSIR, New Delhi.
15. Pharmacographia Indica. 3 Vols. W. Dymock. Reprinted by Bishen Singh Mahendra Pal Singh, Dehradun.
16. Commercial Drugs of India. Dutt, N B. 1980. Reprinted by M/s. Bishen Singh Mahendra Pal Singh, Dehradun.
17. A Dictionary of the Economic Products of India. Watt, G. 6 Vols. 1972. Reprinted by Bishen Singh Mahendra Pal Singh, Dehradun.
18. The Indian Materia Medica. Nadkarni, K. M. 1954. Revised and Enlarged by A. K. Nadkarni. 1972. 2 Vols.
19. Advances in Research in Indian Medicine. Udupa, K. N. et. al., (Eds.). 1970. BHU, Varanasi.
20. All India Consultive Meet on Medicinal and Aromatic Plants. Bangalore, February. 23-25. 1994. Report by Farmer's Development Agency, Chikballapur, Karnataka.

21. Ayurvedic Cure for Common Diseases. Murthy, N. and D. P. Pandey. 1983. Orient Paperbacks, New Delhi.
22. Ayurvedic Cures for Common Diseases. Dash Bhagwan. 1993. Hind Pocket Books Pvt. Ltd. New Delhi.
23. Ayurvedic Drugs and Their Plant Sources. Sivrajan, V. V. and Indira Balachandran. 1994. Oxford and IBH Publishing Co. Pvt. Ltd. Delhi.
24. Ayurvedic Flora Medica. Mooss, N. S. 1978. Vaidyasarathy Press (P) Ltd., Kottayam.
25. Ayurvedic Formulary of India. 2 Parts. 1978. Controller of Publications, Ministry of Health and Family Planning. New Delhi.
26. Ayurvedic Pharmacopoeia of India. Vol. I., Part. I. Controller of Publications, Ministry of Health and Family Planning. New Delhi.
27. Ayurvedic System of Medicine or an Exposition, in English of Hindu Medicine as occurring in Charaka, Susruta, Vagbhatta and other Authoritative Sanskrit Works. Ancient and Modern. Sengupta, Kaviraj Nagendra Nath. 1994. pp. 408. Vol. I and pp. 778. Vol. II. Logos Press, Delhi.
28. Bibliography of Investigated Indian Medicinal Plants. Iyenger, M. A. 1950-1975. M. A. Iyenger Kasturba Medical College, Manipal.
29. Bibliography on Pharmacognosy of Medicinal Plants. Roma Mitra. 1985. National Botanical Research Institute. Botany Information Service, Lucknow.
30. Bombay Materia Medica and Their Therapeutics. Khory, R. N. 1986. Periodical Expert Book Agency, Delhi.
31. Charaka Samhita (A Scientific Synopsis). Ray, P and N. Hirendra. 1980. Indian National Science Academy, Delhi.
32. Catalogue of Indian Synonyms of the Medicinal Plants, Products, Inorganic Substances Etc. Proposed to be included in The Pharmacopoeia of India. Sheriff, M. 1978. Periodical Expert Book Agency. Delhi.
33. CDRI: R and D Highlights. 1951-1990. Central Drug Research Institute, Lucknow.
34. Chemistry and Pharmacology of Ceylon and Indian Medicinal Plants. Chandrasena, J. P. C. 1935. Lucy Chandrasena, Colombo. Sri Lanka.
35. Chemistry of Medicinal Plants. Vol. I. 1993. Central Council for Research in Unani Medicine, Delhi.
36. Clinical Application of Ayurvedic Remedies and a List of Ayurvedic Preparations. 1986. Sri Satguru Publications, Delhi.
37. Commercial Products of India Being an Abridgment of the Dictionary of the Economic Products of India. George, W. Repr. 1966. Today and Tommorrow's Printers and Publishers. Delhi.
38. Companion to Chopra's Glossary of Indian Medicinal Plants. Mehrotra, B. N. et. al., 1987. Bishen Singh Mahendra Pal Singh, Dehradun.
39. Comparative Hindu Materia Medica. Chakraberty, C. Repr. 1983. Neeraj Publishing House, Delhi.
40. Compendium of Indian Medicinal Plants. Mehrotra, B. N. and R. P. Rastogi. 1990-1993. Vols. 1-3. Central Drug Research Institute and Publications & Information Directorate (CSI(R) Lucknow and Delhi.
41. Cultivation and Utilization of Aromatic Plants. Atal, C. K. and B. M. Kapur (Eds.) 1982. Regional Research Laboratory (CSIR), Jammu Tawi. Vol. I and II.

42. Current Research on Medicinal Plants in India. Dhawan, B. N. (Ed.) 1986. Indian National Science Academy, Delhi.
43. Dictionary of Economic Plants in India. Singh, Umrao et. al., 1983. Indian Council of Agricultural Research, Delhi.
44. Dictionary of Indian Medicinal Plants. Husain, Akhtar. et. al., 1992. Central Institute of Medicinal & Aromatic Plants. Lucknow.
45. Distribution of British Pharmacopoeial Drug Plants and Their Subsitutes Growing in India. Nayar, S. L. and I. C. Chopra. 1992. CSIR, New Delhi.
46. Encyclopaedia of Indian Medicine Vol. I. Ramachandra Rao, S. K. (Ed.). 1985. Popular Prakashan Pvt. Ltd. Bombay.
47. Everybody's Guide to Ayurvedic Medicine. Dastur, J. F. 1978. D. B. Taraporevala Sons & Co. (P) Ltd. Bombay.
48. Flora Medica: A Botanical Account of All the More Important Plants Used in Medicine. Lindley, John. Repr. 1981. Ajay Books Service. Delhi.
49. Fundamentals of Ayurvedic Medicine. Dash Bhagwan. 1989. Konark Publishers (P) Ltd. and Bansal & Co. Delhi.
50. Glossary of Indian Medicinal Plants. Chopra, R. N. et. al., Repr. 1989. CSIR, New Delhi.
51. Glossary of Indian Medicinal Plants with Active Principles, Second Supplement. Part. I. A – K. Asolkar, L. V. et. al., 1992 (1965-1991). CSIR. Publications & Information Directorate, Delhi.
52. Glossary of Indian Medicinal Plants. Supplement. Chopra, R. N. et. al., 1969. CSIR. Publications & Information Directorate, Delhi.
53. Glossary of Vegetable Drugs in Brhattrayi. Singh T. B. and K. C. Chunekar. 1972. Chowkhamba Sanskrit Series Office, Varanasi.
54. Glossary of Vegetable Drugs in Vagbhatta. Godbole, S. R. et. al., 1966. Indian Drugs Research Association. Pune.
55. Handbook of Ayurveda. Dash, Bhagwan & Junius, Manfred M. Repr. 1987. Concept Publishing Company, Delhi.
56. Handbook of Ayurvedic Medicinal Plants. Kapoor, L. D. 1990. CRC Press, Boca Raton, USA.
57. Handbook of Medicinal Plants. Kurup, P. N. V. et. al. Rev. and Enlarged ed. 1980. Central Council for Research in Ayurveda & Siddha, Delhi.
58. Herbal Drugs in Indian Pharmaceutical Industry. Kapoor, S. L. & R. Mitra. 1979. NBRI. Economic Botany Information Service, Lucknow.
59. Herbal Formulary of Essential Drugs of Ayurveda. Chunekar, K. C. & V. K. Joshi. 1988. World Health Organization, Kathmandu (Nepal).
60. Illustraded Materia Medica of Indo-Tibetan Medicine. Dash Bhagwan. 1987. Classics India Publications, Delhi.
61. Indian Materia Medica with Ayurvedic, Unnani-Tibbi, Siddha, Allopathic, Homoeopathic, Naturopathic and Home Remedies, Appendices and Indexes. Vols. I and II. Nadkarni, K. M. 3 rd rev. and enl. edn. Popular Book Depot & Dhootapapeshwar Prakashan. Vol. I and II.
62. Indian Medicinal Plants. A Compedium of 500 species. Arya Vaidya Sala. 1996. 5 vols. Orient Longman Ltd. Delhi.
63. Indigenous Drugs of India. Chopra, R. N. et. al., 2 nd rev. and enl. edn. 1982. Academic Publishers, Delhi.
64. International Workshop on Tissue Culture & Biotechnology of Medicinal & Aromatic Plants. Lucknow. December 14-16. 1987. Central Institute of Medicinal & Aromatic Plants.

65. Materia Indica. 2 vols. Ainslie, Whitelaw. Repr. 1984. Neeraj Publishing House, Delhi.

66. Materia Medica. 2 vols. Honigberger, John Martin. Repr. 1986. B. R. Publishing Corporation, Delhi.

67. Materia Medica of Ayurveda Based on Ayurveda Saukhyam of Todarananda. Dash Bhagwan. 1980. Concept Publishing Company, Delhi.

68. Materia Medica of Ayurveda Based on Madanpala's Nighantu. Dash Bhagwan. Repr. 1994. B. Jain Publishers (P) Ltd. Delhi.

69. Materia Medica of India and Their Therapeutics. Khory Rustomjee Naserwanjee & Katrak, Nanabhai Navrosji. Repr. 1981. Neeraj Publishing House, Delhi.

70. Medical and Economic Aspects of Some Indian Medicinal Plants. Chopra, R. N. 1932. Patna University, Patna.

71. Medicinal and Poisonous Plants of India. Caius, J. F. 1986. Scientific Publishers, Jodhpur.

72. Medicinal Chemistry Research in India. Singh, H. et. al., 1985. CDRI. National Information Centre for Drugs & Pharmaceuticals, Lucknow.

73. Medicinal Flora of India. Duke, James. 1981. Economic Botany Laboratory, USA.

74. Medicinal Plants and Their Cultivation. Husain, Akhtar. 1993. CIMAP, Lucknow.

75. Medicinal Plants of India. Jain, S. K. and De. Filipps, R. A. 1991. Reference Publications Inc., Algonac, Michigan (US(A)

76. Medicinal Plants of India. Vol. 1 : A – G; Vol. 2 : H – P. 1976 & 1987. Satyavati, G. V. et. al., Indian Council of Medical Research, Delhi.

77. Medicinal Plants of India and Pakistan. Dastur, J. F. 1977. D. B. Taraporevala Sons & Co. (P) Ltd. Bombay.

78. Medicinal Plants. Bibliography of CSIR Contributions. 1950-1997. Ambasta, S. P. CSIR. CSIR. Publications & Information Directorate, Delhi.

79. Medicinal Plants: New Vistas of Research. Govil, J. N. et. al., 1993. Part 1 and Part 2. Today & Tomorrow's Printers & Publishers, Delhi.

80. Pharmacognosy. Kokate, C. K. et. al., 1990. Nirali Prakashan, Pune.

81. Pharmacognosy of Ayurvedic Drugs- Kerala. Series 1 – 9. Published by Central Research Institute of the Former Travancore University.

82. Pharmacognosy of Indian Leaf Drugs. Datta, S. C. and Mukerji, B. Govt. of India Press, Calcutta.

83. Pharmacognosy of Indian Root and Rhizome Drugs. Datta, S. C. and B. Mukerji. Manager of Publications. Govt. of India Press, Calcutta.

84. Pharmacographia: A History of the Principal Drugs of Vegetable Origin Met With in Great Britain and British India. Flueckiger, Friedrich, A. and Daniel Hanbury. Repr. 1986. International Book Distributors, Dehradun.

85. Pharmacopoeia Indica, Being a Collection of Vegetable, Mineral and Animal Drugs in Common Use in India. Bose, Kartick. C. Repr. 1984. Bishen Singh Mahendra Pal Singh, Dehradun.

86. Pharmacopoeia of India. Ministry of Health and Family Welfare. Controller of Publications, Delhi. III rd edn. 1985.

87. Pharmacopoeial Standards for Ayurvedic Formulations. Central Council for Research in Ayurveda & Siddha, Delhi. 1987.
88. Phytochemical Investigations of Certain Medicinal Plants Used in Ayurveda. Pandey, V. N. (Ed.) Central Council for Research in Ayurveda and Siddha, Delhi. 1990.
89. Poisonous plants of India. Chopra, R. N. et. al., Indian Council of Agricultural Research, Delhi. 1984.
90. Recent Advances in Medicinal, Aromatic and Spice Crops. 2 Vols. Raychaudhuri, S. P. (Ed.) Today & Tomorrow's Printers & Publishers, Delhi. 1991.
91. Report on Propagation Methods of Medicinal Plants of India – I. Tropical Botanic Garden & Research Institute and Lok Swasthya Parampar Samvardhan Samiti, Thiruvananthapuram and Coimbatore.
92. Review of Research on Indian Medicinal and Allied Plants. Chopra, I. C. and K. L. Handa. ICAR Review Series, 34. Indian Council of Agricultural Research, Delhi.
93. Review of Work on Indian Medicinal Plants (Including Indigenous Drugs and Poisonous Plants). Chopra, R. N. & Chopra, I. C. ICMR Special Report Series, 30. Indian Council of Medical Research, Delhi.
94. Single Drug Remedies with Illustrations. Mooss, N. S. Vaidyasarathy Press (P) Ltd., Kottayam. 1976.
95. Some controversial Drugs in Indian Medicine. Bapalal Vaidya. Chaukhambha Orientalia, Varanasi. 1982. Jaikrishnadas Ayurveda Series, 33.
96. Speaking of Ayurvedic Remedies for Common Diseases. Devaraj, T. L. Sterling Publishers (P) Ltd, Delhi. Rev. edn. 1994.
97. Studies on Medicinal Plants in Dhanvantariya Nighantu Vol. I. Kamat, D. K. & S. D. Mahajan (Eds.) 1972. Published by Kamat Publishers. 18 Rasta Peth, Pune.
98. Studies on Pharmacognosy of Some Indian Medicinal Plants. Deshmukh, V. K. et. al., IDRA Publications, I. Published by Indian Drug Research Association, Pune.
99. Subsitute and Adulterant Plants. Garg, Sunita. Periodical Expert Book Agency, Delhi. 1992.
100. Susruta Samhita, a Scientific Synopsis. Ray, Priyadaranjan et al., Indian National Science Academy, Delhi. 1980.
101. Therapeutic Guide to Ayurvedic Medicine (a Handbook on Ayurvedic Medicine). Pathak, Ram, R. Baidyanath Ayurved Bhawan Ltd. Patna. 1970.
102. Treatise on Indian Medicinal Plants. Vol – I. Chatterjee, Asima & Pakrashi, Satyesh Chandra. 1991. Council of Scientific & Industrial Research. Publications & Information Directorate, Delhi.
103. Ultraviolet and Visible Spectra of Herbal Drugs. Shafiullah, A. M. Aligarh Muslim University Press, Aligarh. 1992.
104. Useful Plants of India. Ambasta, S. P. (Ed.) Council of Scientific & Industrial Research. Publications & Information Directorate, Delhi. Repr. 1992.

105. Useful Plants of India; with Notices of Their Chief Value in Commerce, Medicine and the Arts. Drury, Heber. Repr. 1978. International Book Distributors and Periodical Expert. Book Agency, Dehradun and Delhi.

106. Vegetable Materia Medica of India and Ceylon. Roberts Emmanuel. Bishen Singh Mahendra Pal Singh, Dehradun. Repr. 1984.

107. Wealth of India: A Dictionary of Indian Raw Materials and Industrial Products- Raw Materials. 11 Vols. 2 Suppls. Council of Scientific & Industrial Research, Publications & Information Directorate, Delhi. 1948-1986.

108. Wealth of India: A Dictionary of Indian Raw Materials and Industrial Products – Raw Materials. Council of Scientific & Industrial Research, Publications & Information Directorate, Delhi. 1987 onwards.

109. Workshop on Drug Research in Ayurveda, New Itanagar, May 24-25. 1993. Abstracts. Central Council for Research in Ayurveda & Siddha, Delhi. Sponsored by CCRAS.

110. Workshop on Information Management for the Medicinal & Aromatic Plants Industry, Delhi. October. 12-14. 1993. Report. Jain, H. C. et. al., Council of Scientific & Industrial Research. Publications & Information Directorate, Delhi. Published in 1994.

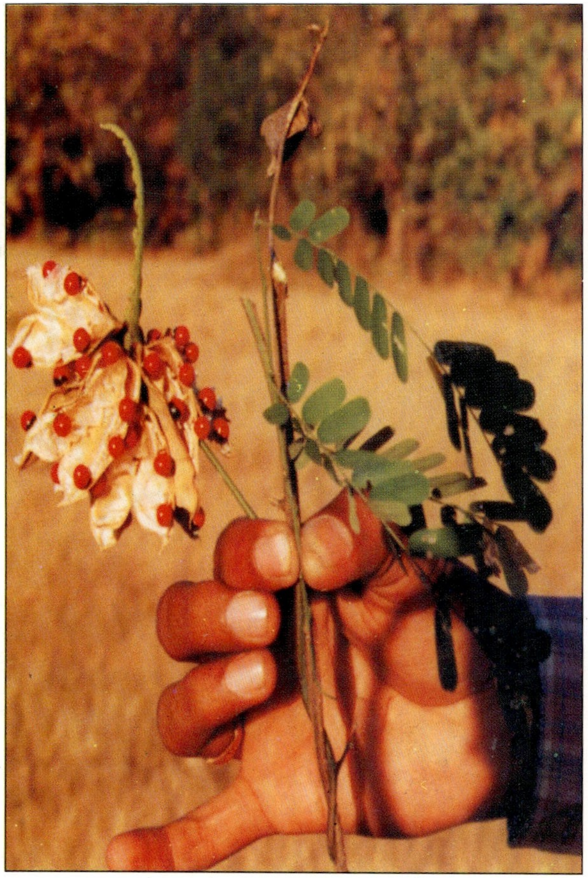

Plate 1. Abrus precatorius L
(Fabaceae)

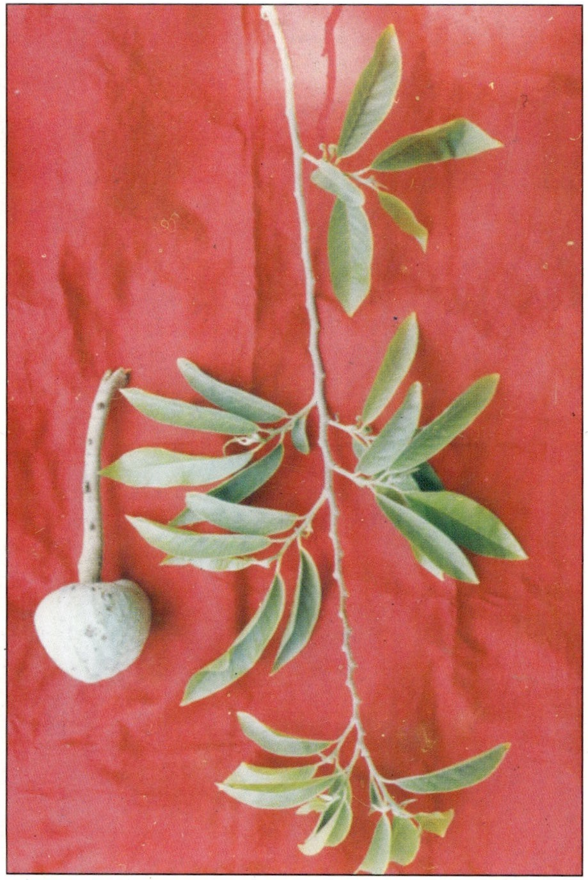

Plate 2. Annona reticulata L
(Annonaceae)

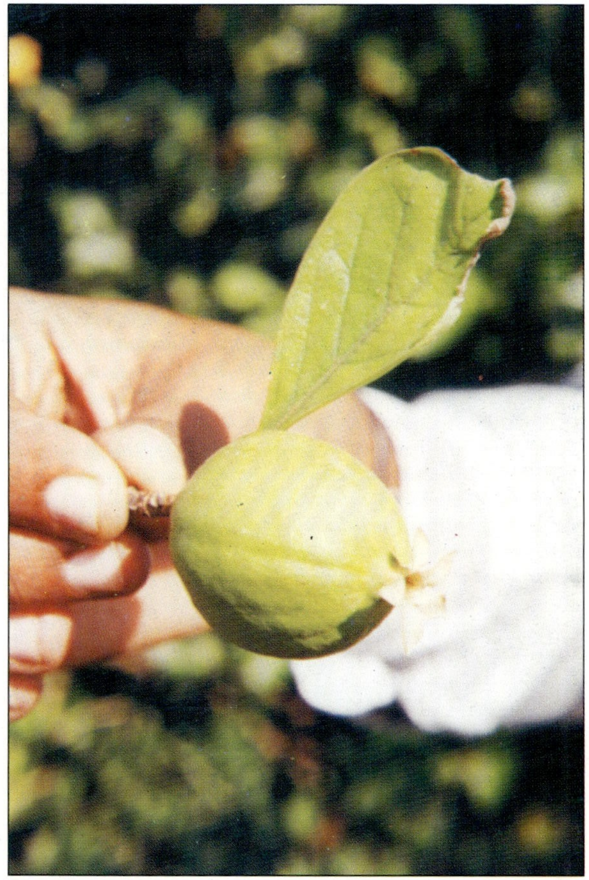

Plate 3. Catunaregam spinosa (Thunb)
Tirvengadum (Rubiaceae)

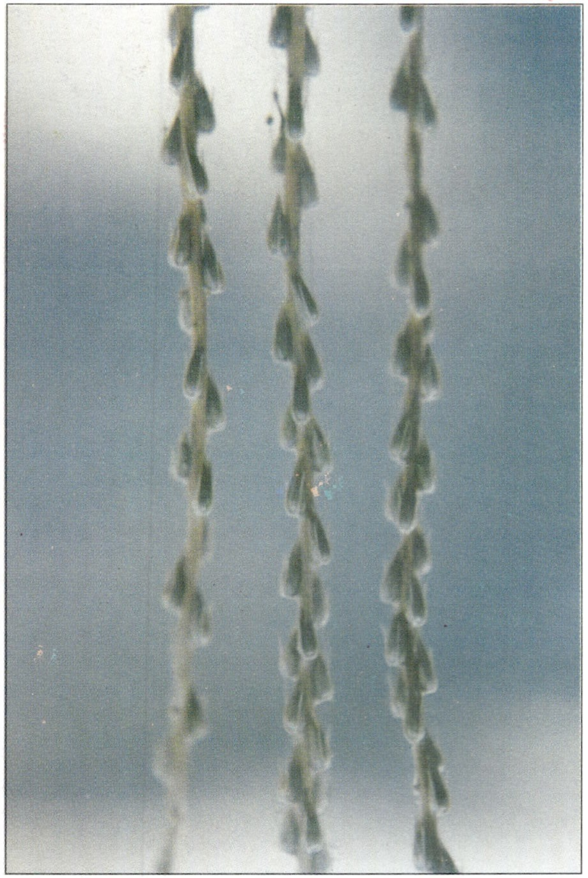

Plate 4. Achyranthes aspera L
(Amaranthaceae)

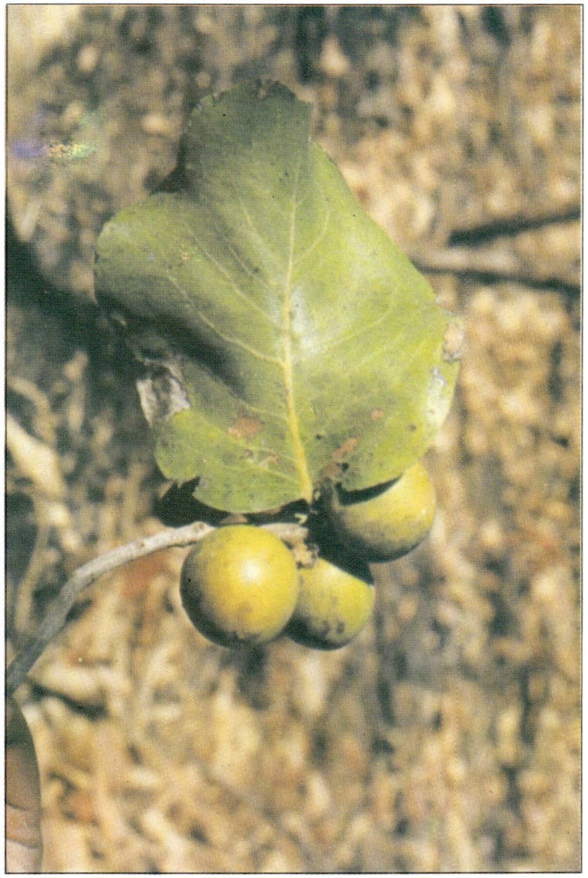

Plate 5. Diospyros melanoxylon Roxb
(Ebenaceae)

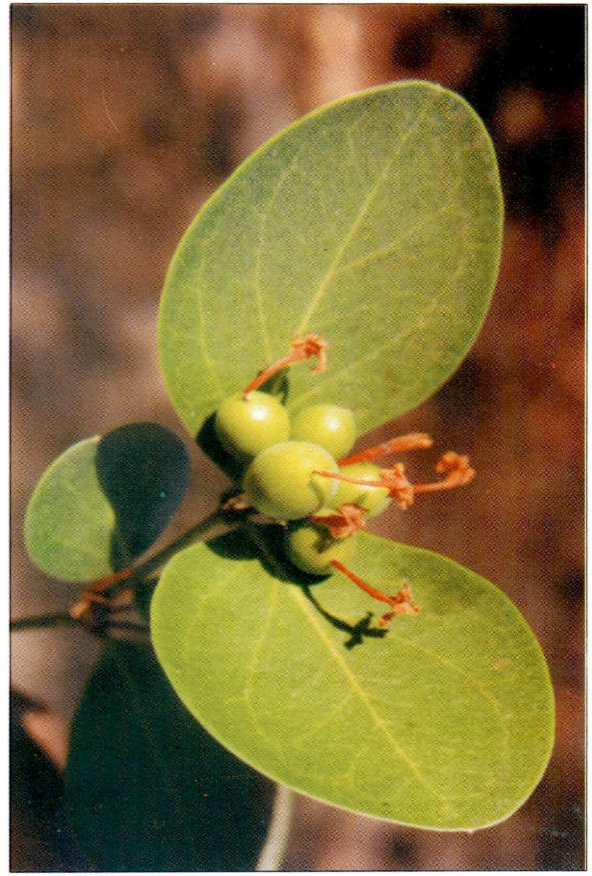

Plate 6. Carissa congesta Wight
(Apocynaceae)

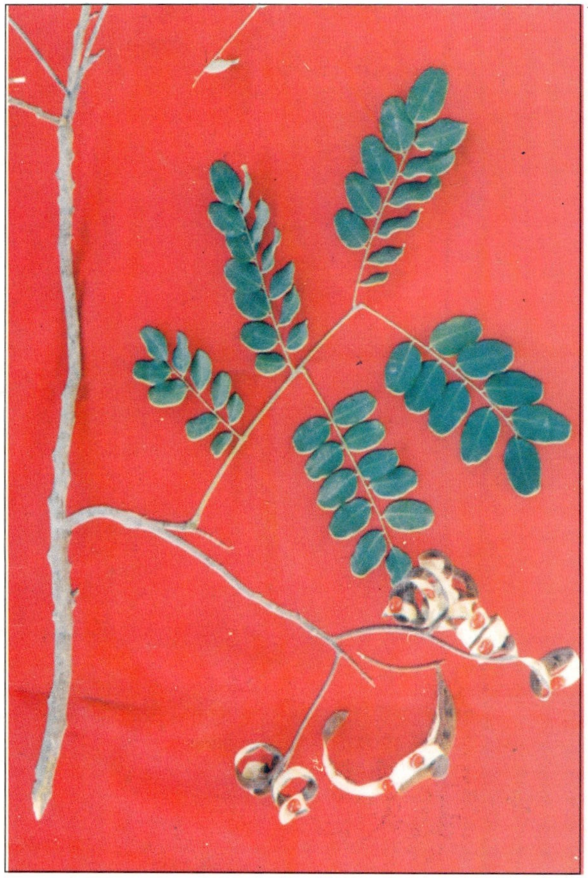

Plate 7. Adenanthera pavonina L
(Mimosaceae)

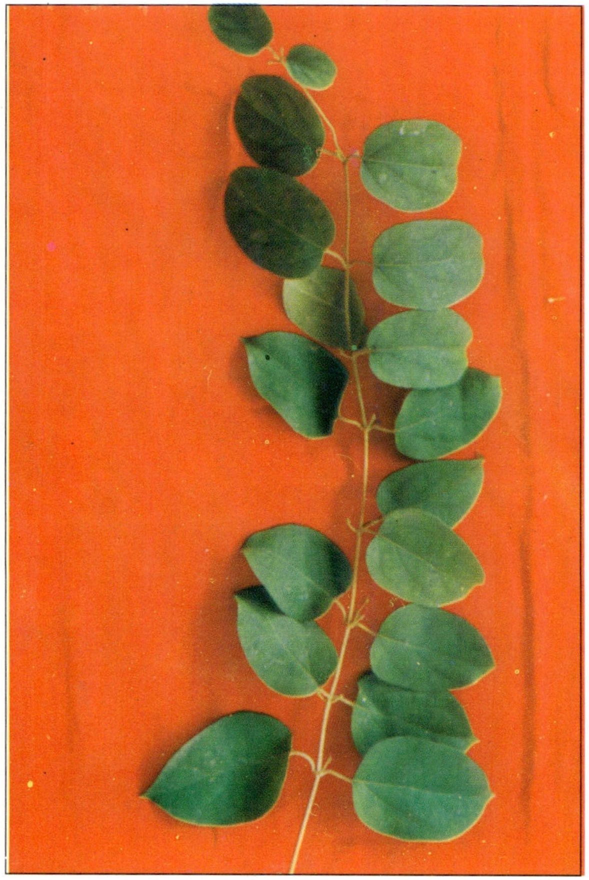

Plate 8. Gymnema sylvestre (Retz) Sm
(Asclepiadaceae)

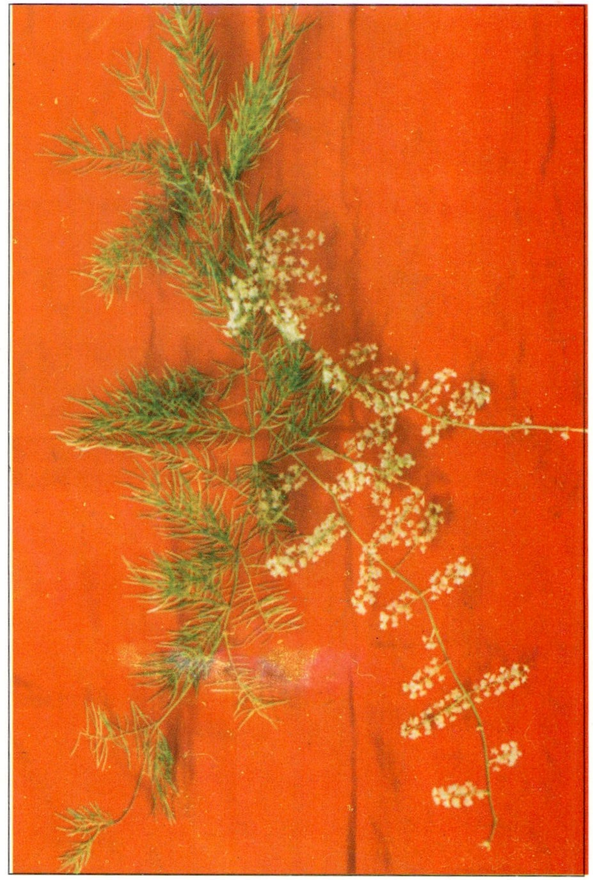

Plate 9. Asparagus racemosus Wild
(Liliaceae)

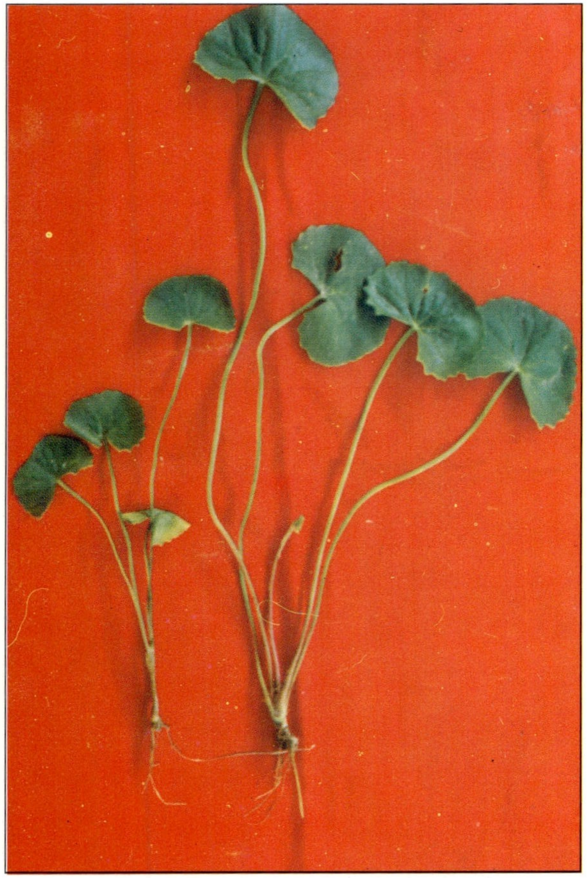

Plate10. Centella asiatica (L) Urb
(Apiaceae)

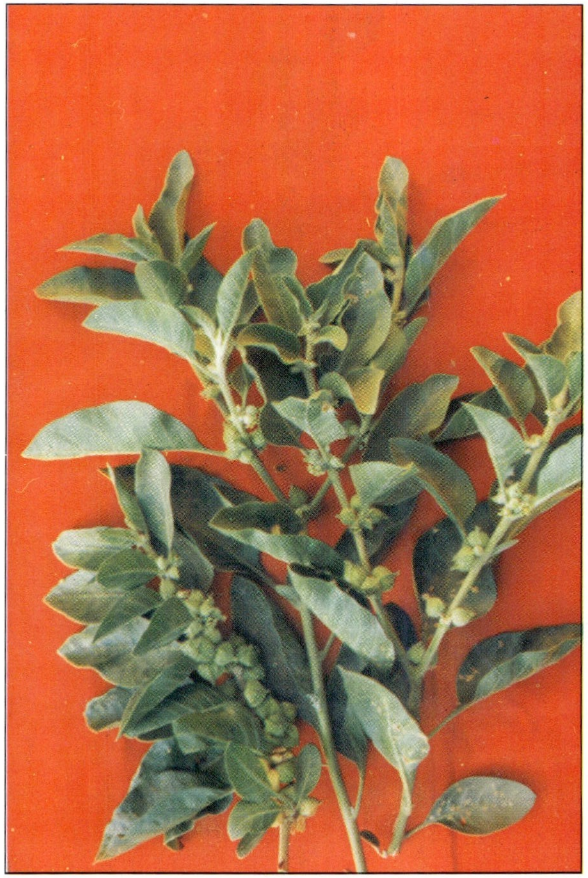

Plate 11. Withania Somnifera (L) Dunal
(Solanaceae)

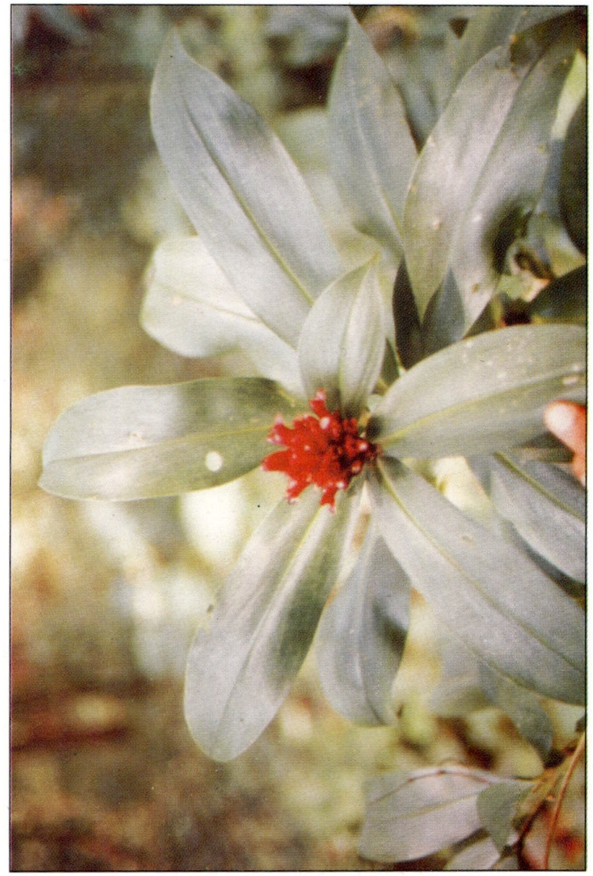

Plate 12. Costus speciosus
(Koening ex Retz)Sm (Zingiberaceae)

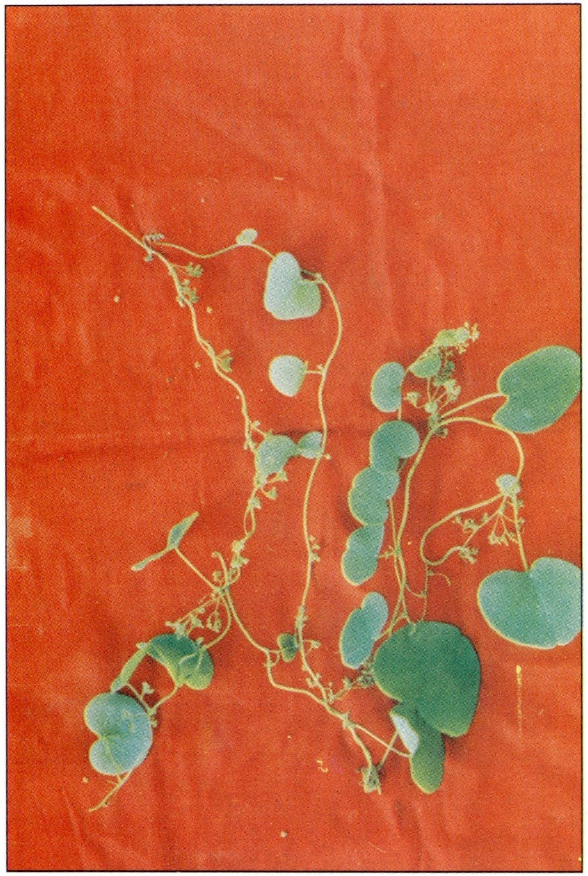

Plate 13. Cissampelos pariera L
(Menispermaceae)

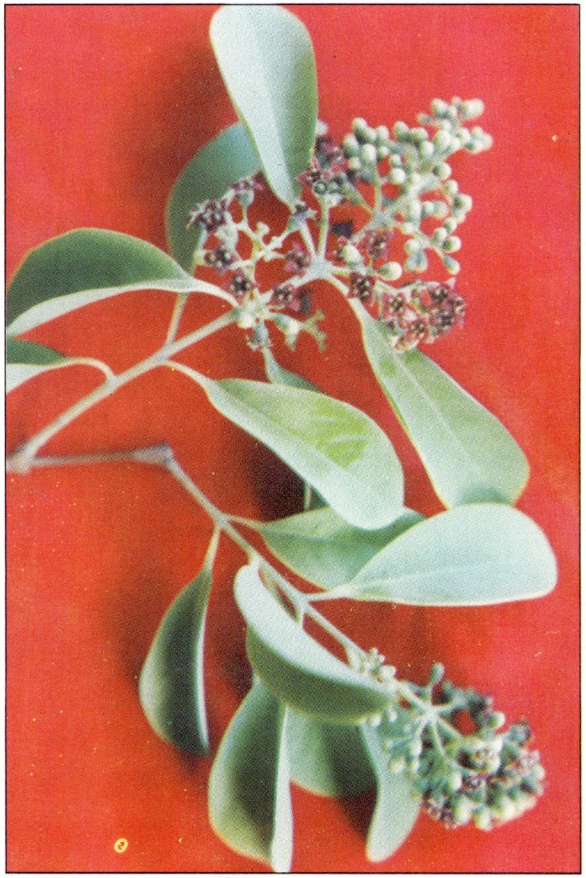

Plate 14. Santalum album L
(Santalaceae)

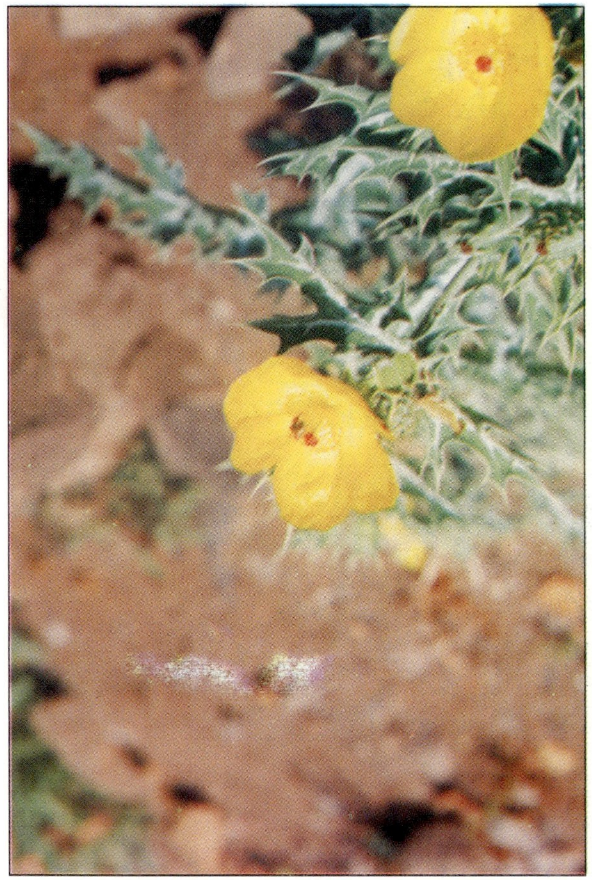

Plate 15. Argemone mexicana L
(Papaveraceae)

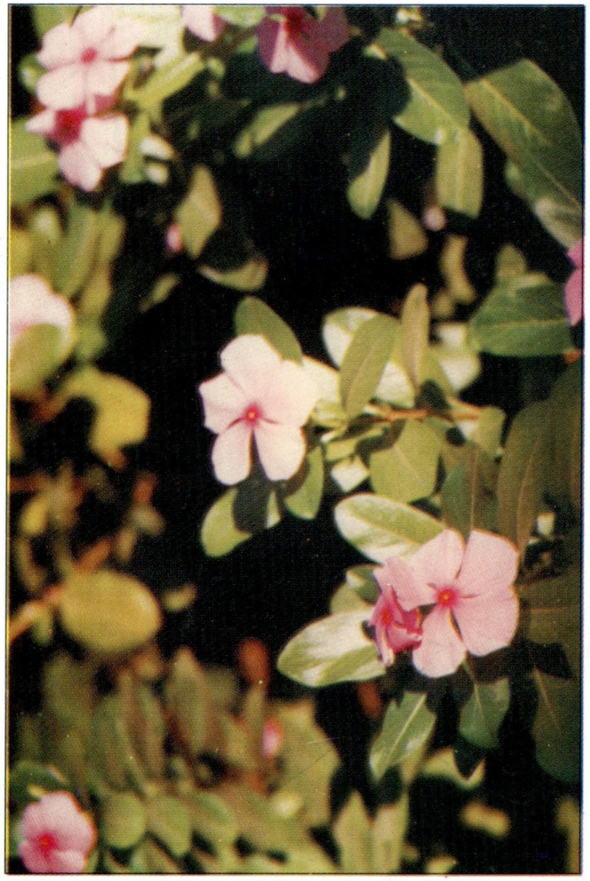

Plate 16. Catharanthus roseus (L) G Don (Apocynaceae)

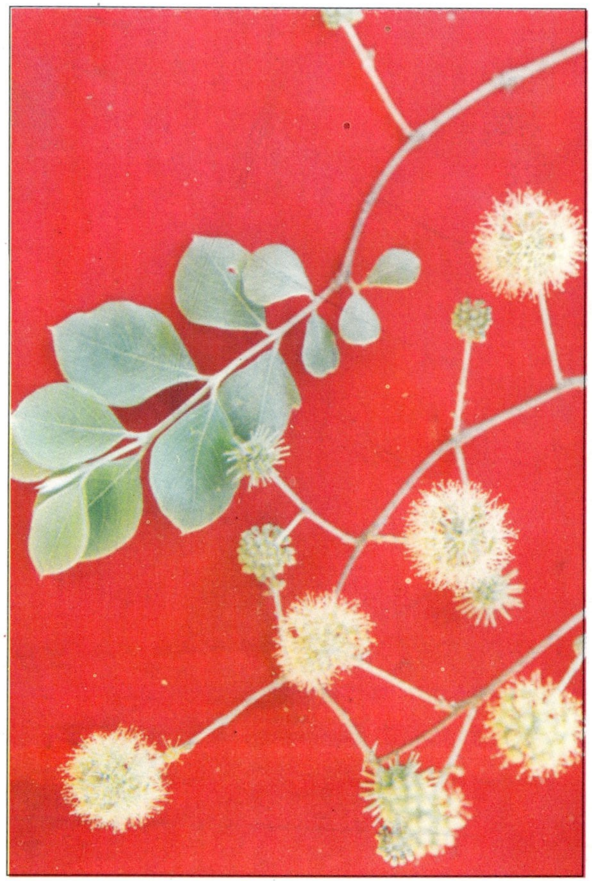

Plate 17. Anogeissus latifolia (Roxb) Wall ex Bedd (Combretaceae)

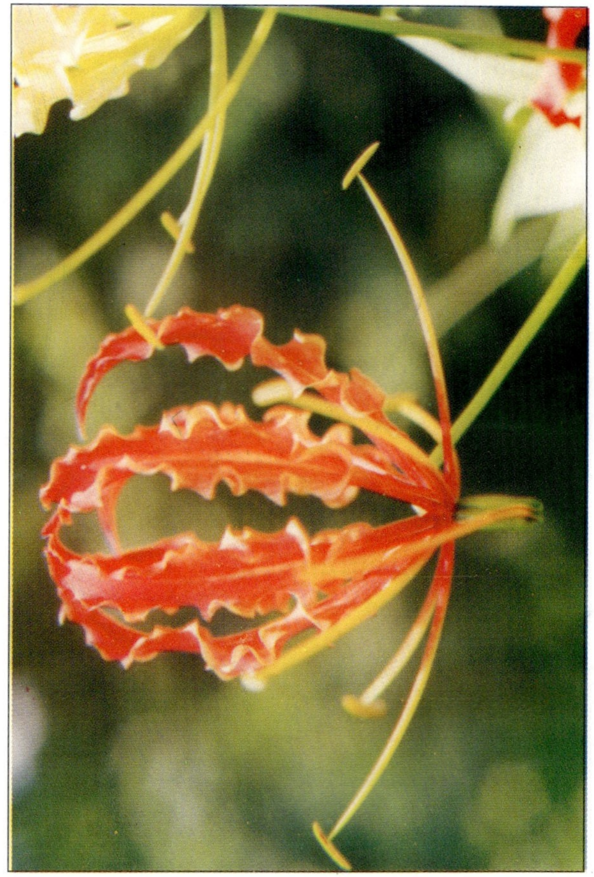

Plate 18. Gloriosa superba L (Liliaceae)

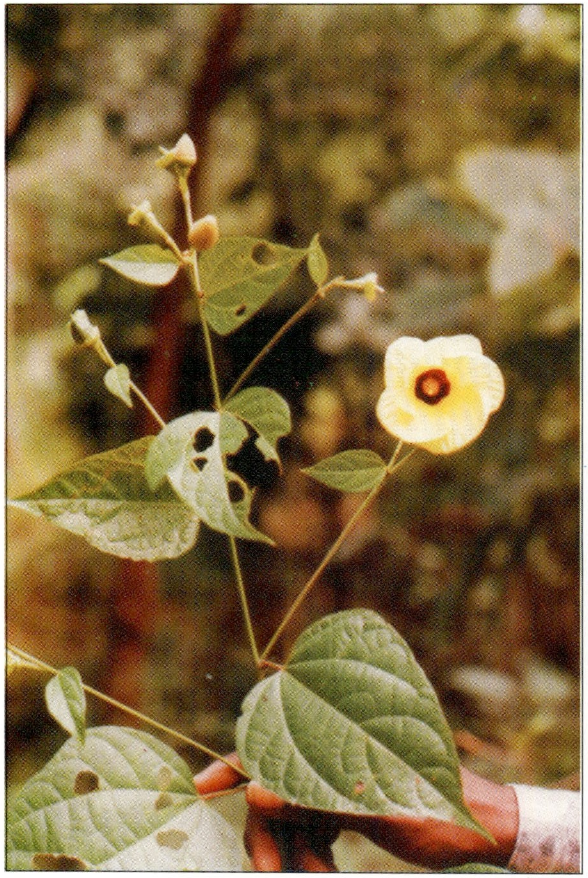

Plate 19. Thespesia lampus (Cav) Dalz & Gibs (Malvaceae)

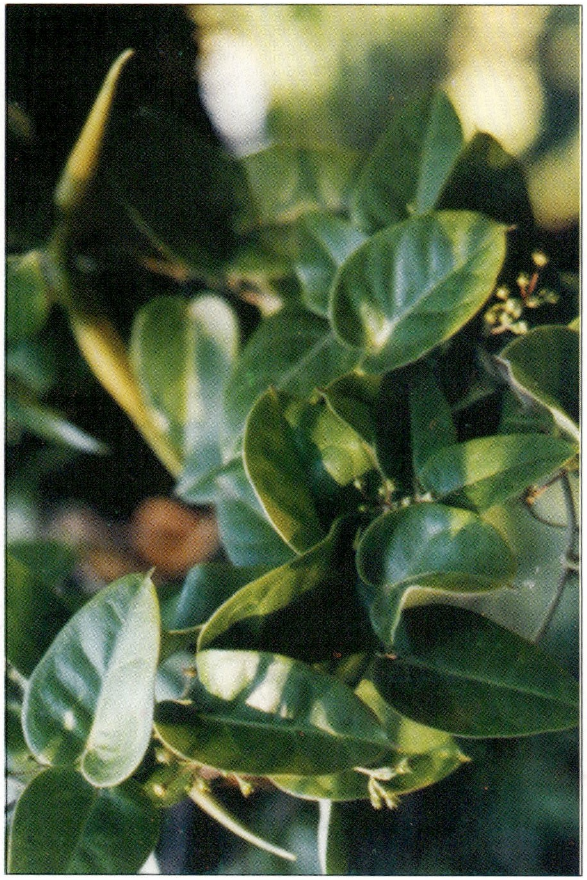

Plate 20. Tylophora indica (Burm F) Merr (Asclepiadaceae)

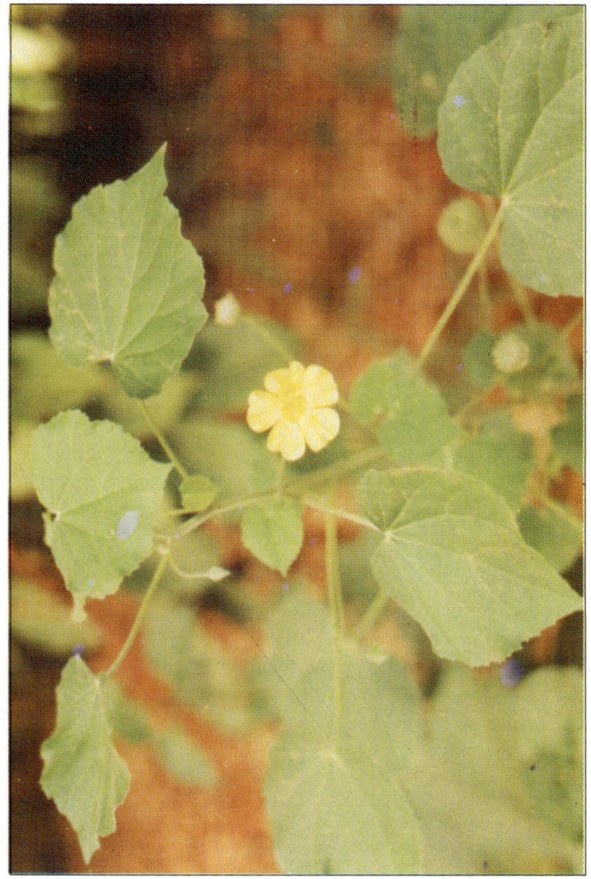

Plate 21. Abutilon indicum L Sw (Malvaceae)

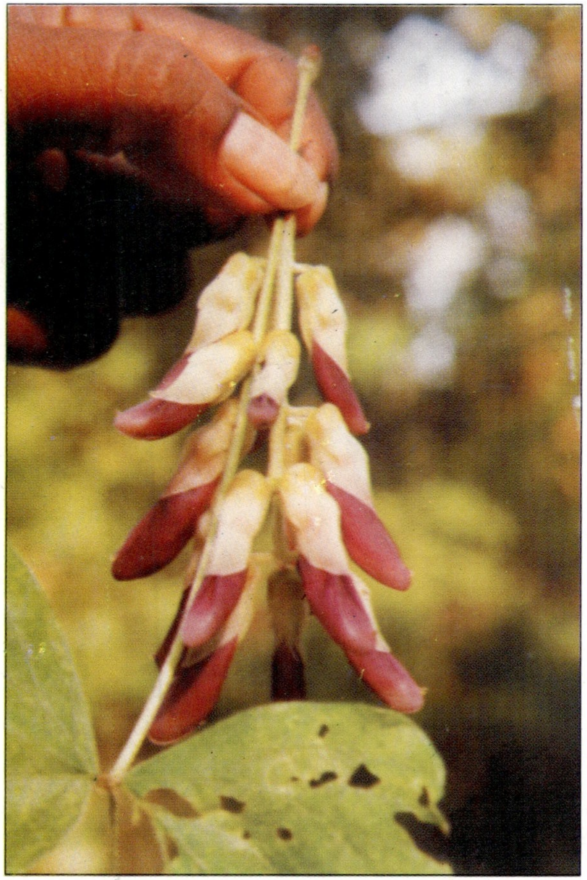

Plate 22. Canavalia gladiata (Jacq) DC
(Fabaceae)

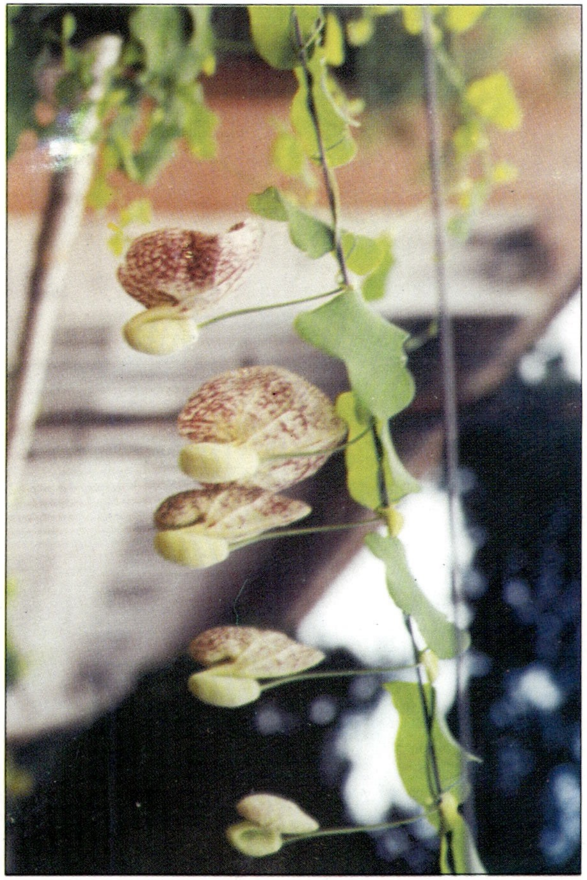

Plate 23. Aristolochia indica L
(Aristolochiaceae)

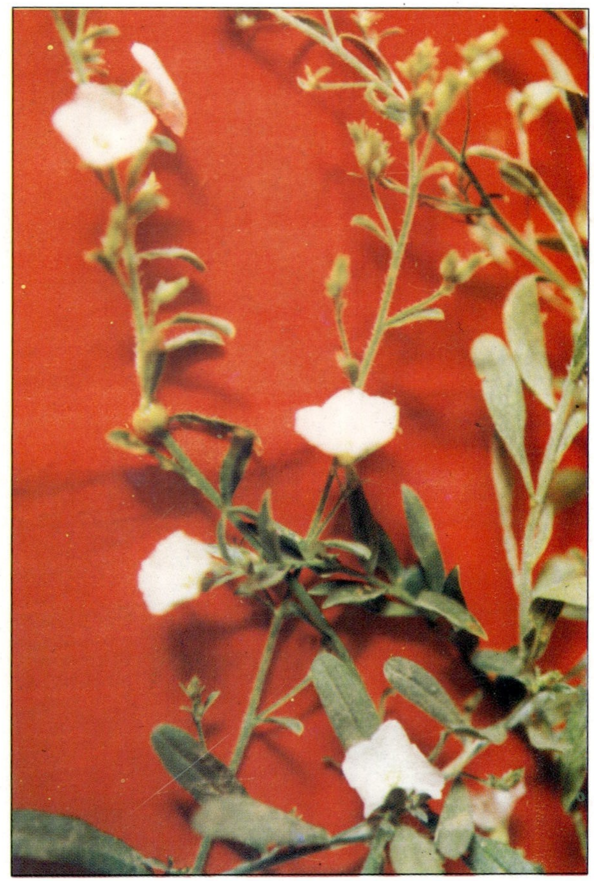

Plate 24. Evolvulus alsinoides L
(Convolvulaceae)